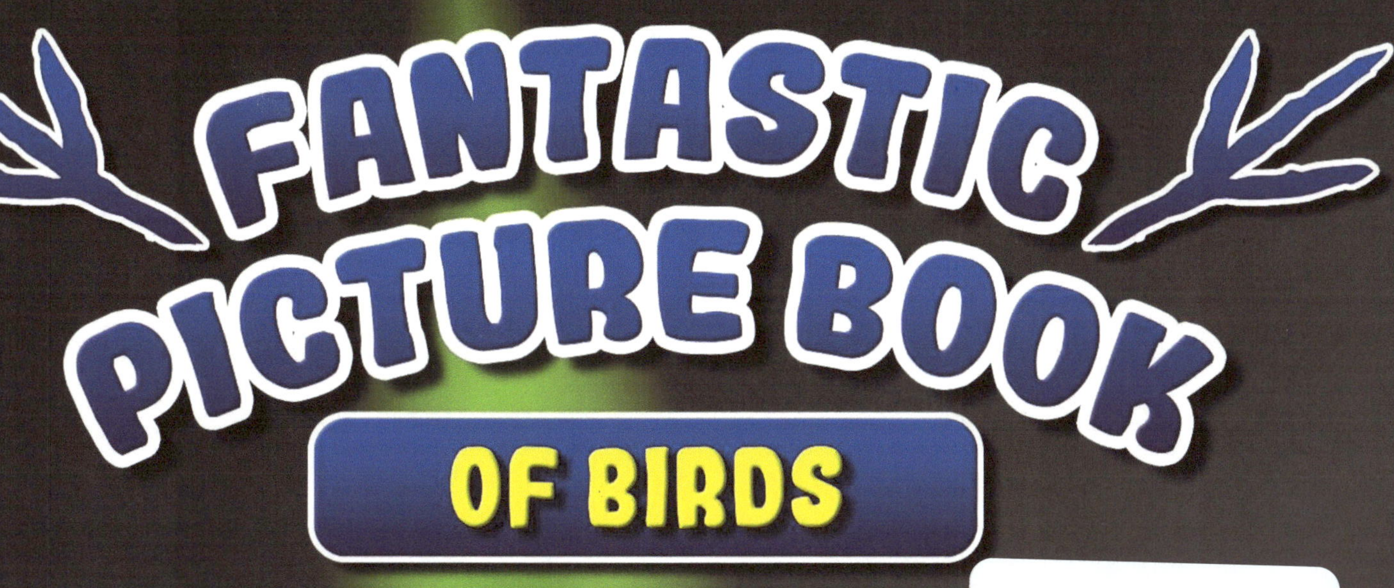

Copyright © Rodrick Madison

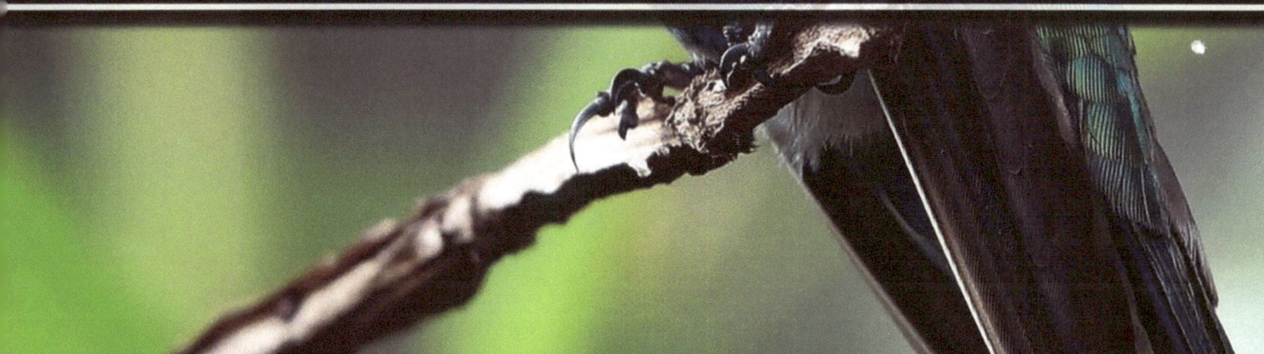

BALD EAGLE

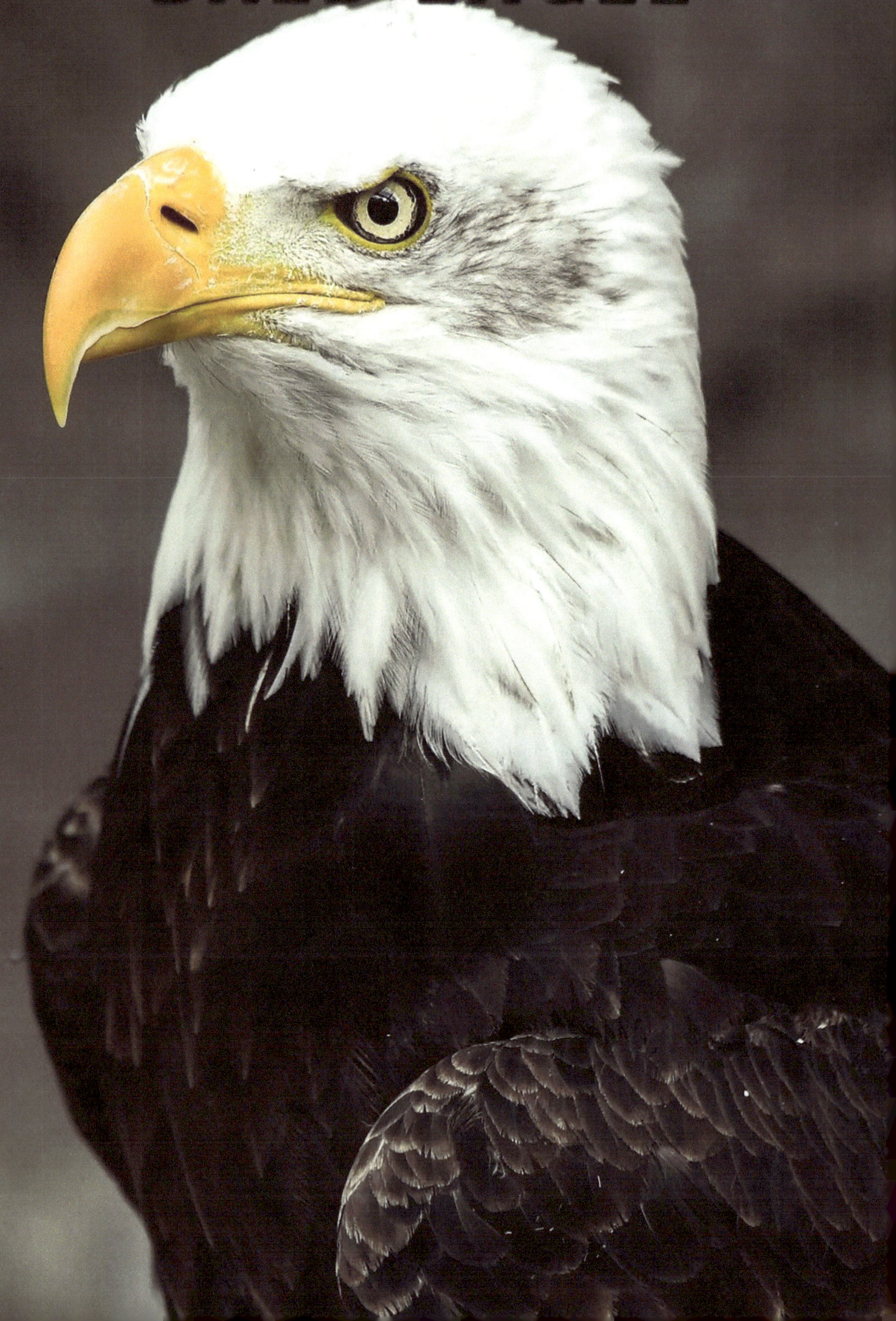

BEE EATERS

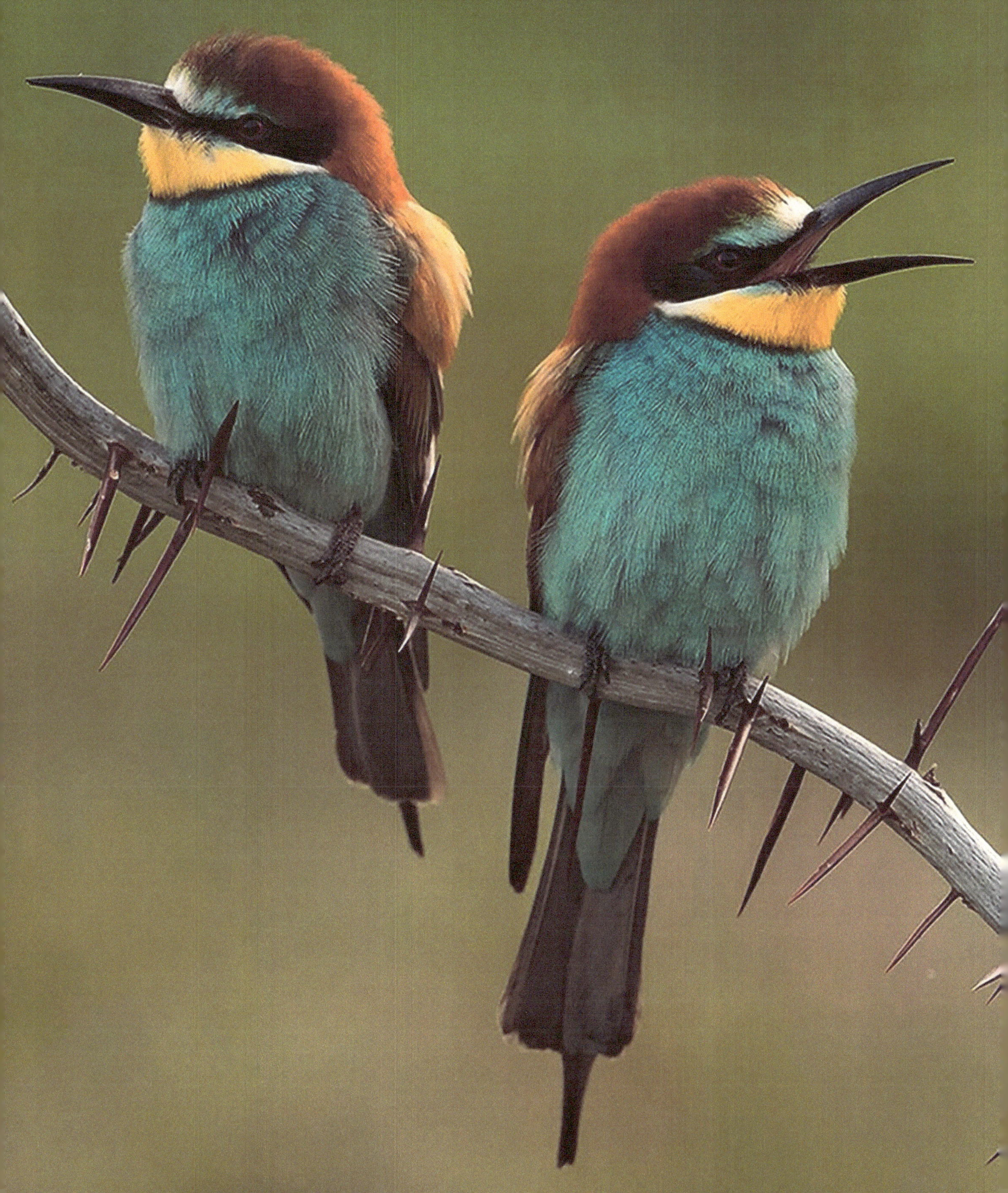

BLACK REDSTART

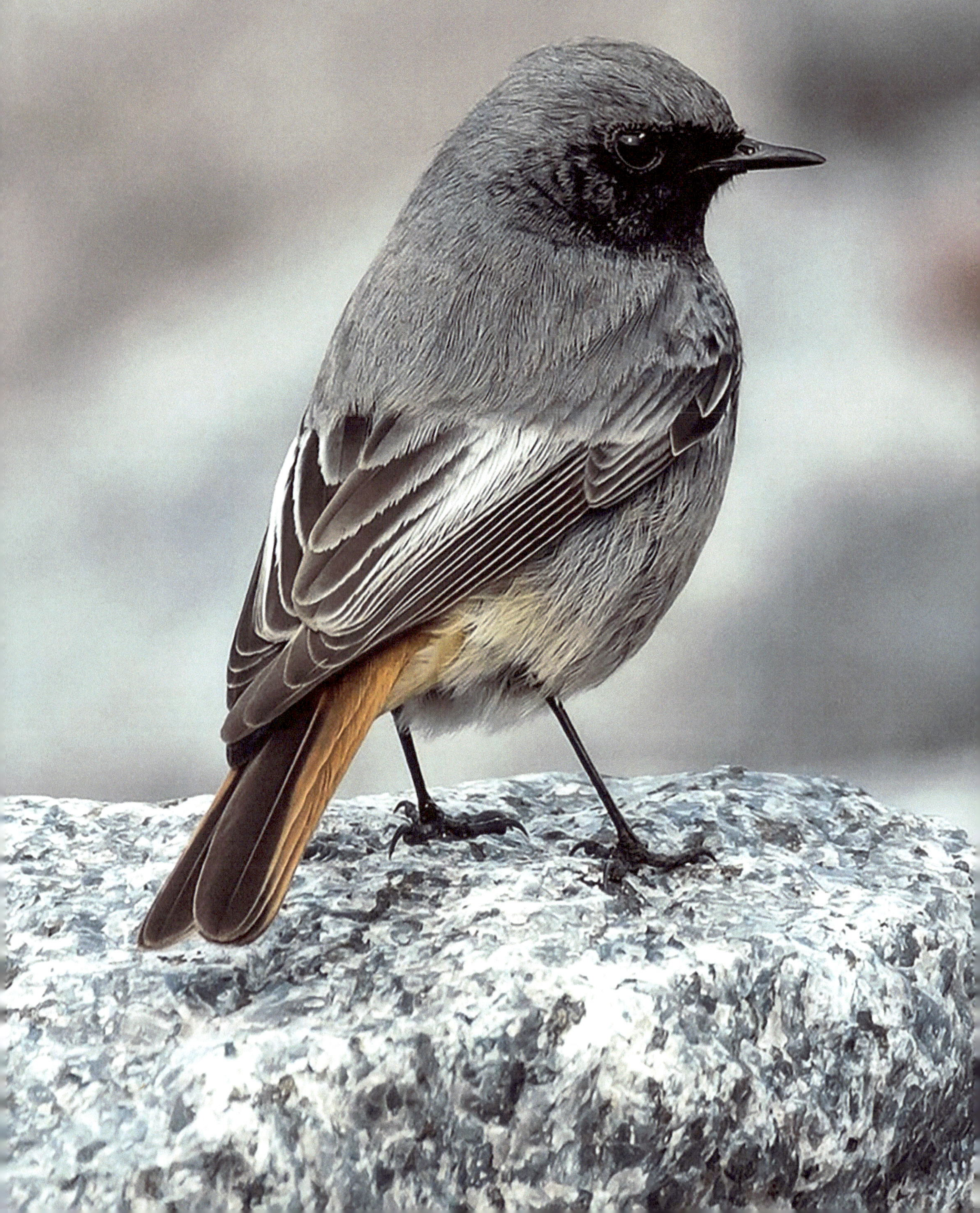

EURASIAN BLUE TIT

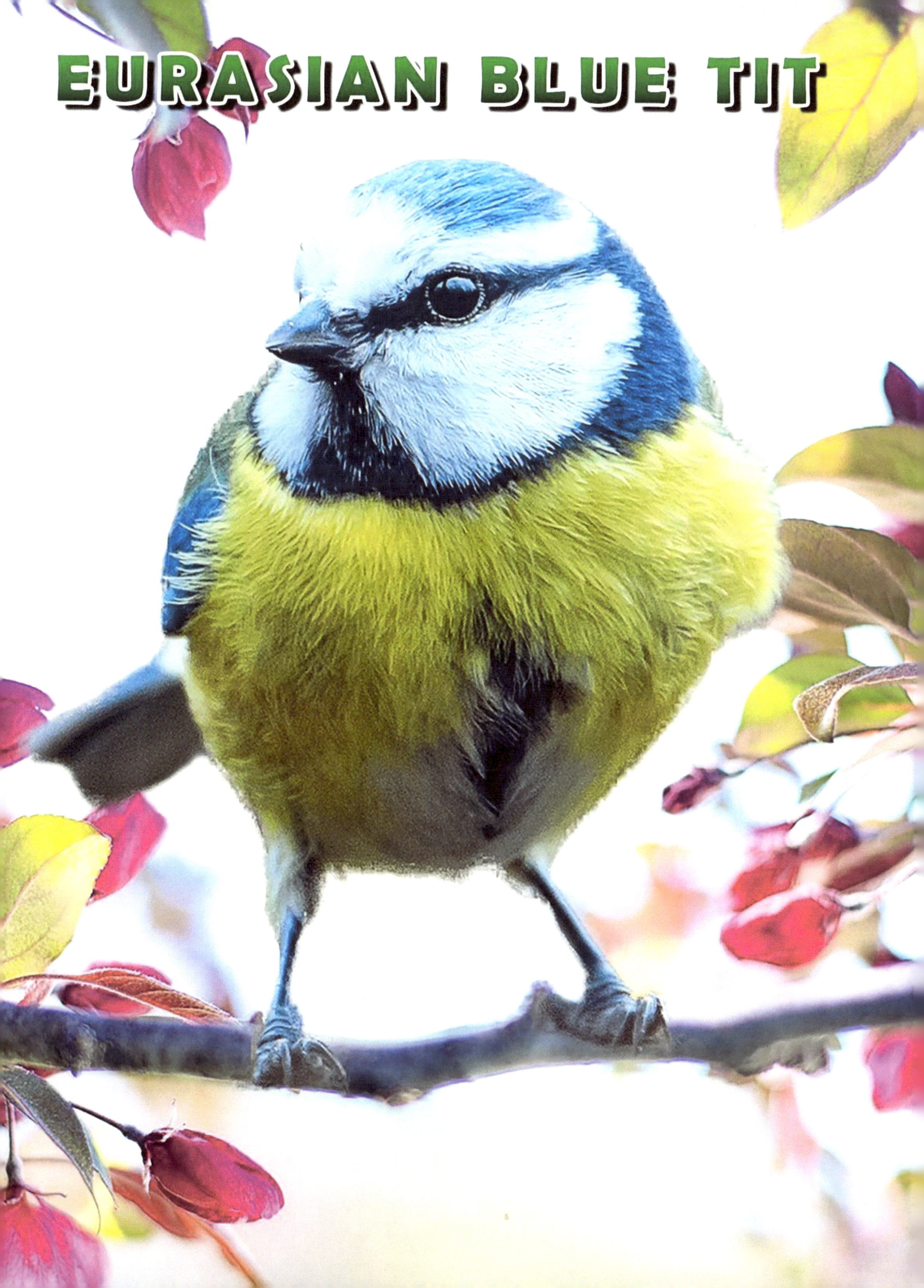

CARDINAL

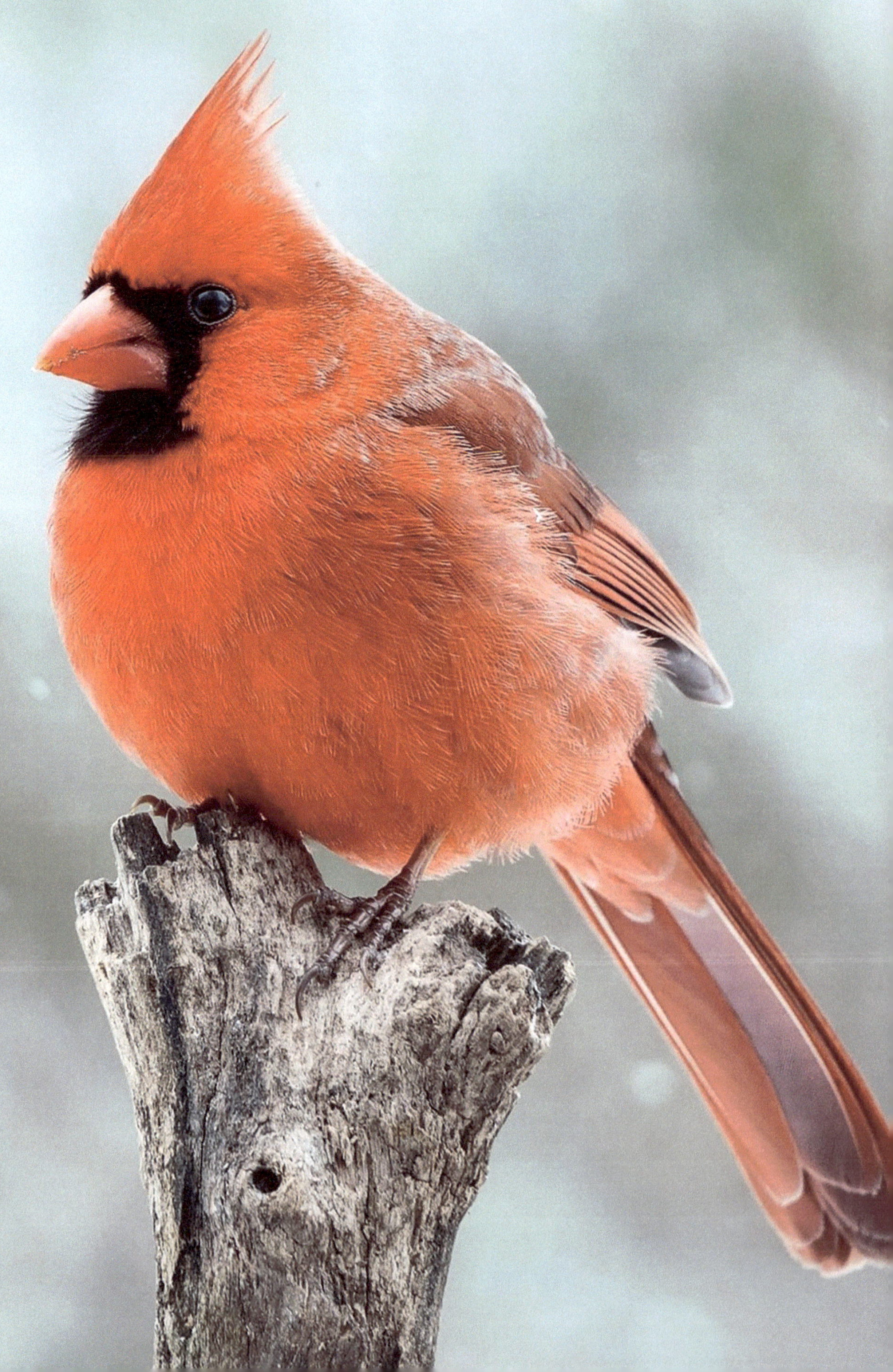

COMMON CHAFFINCH

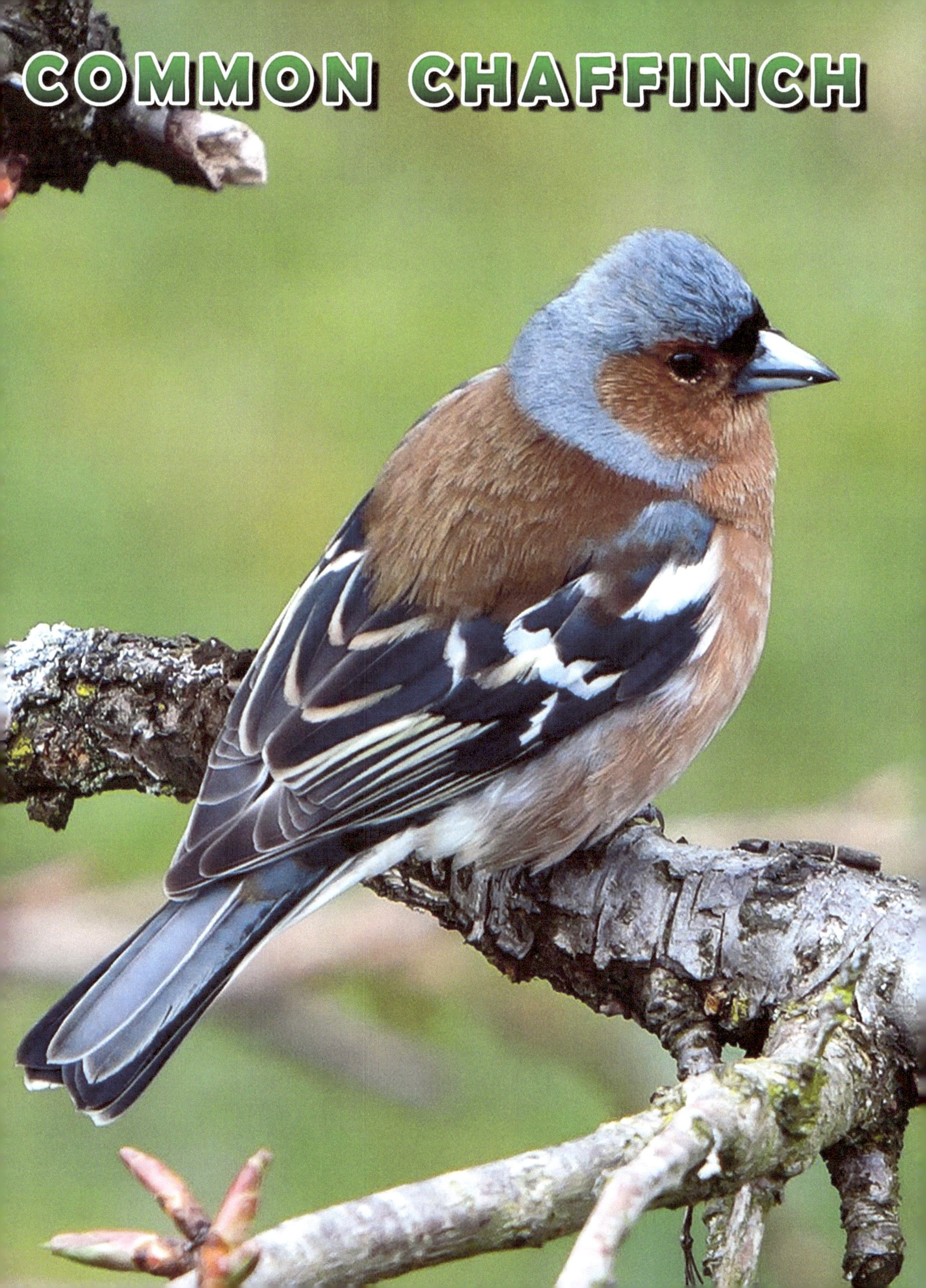

CHICKADEE

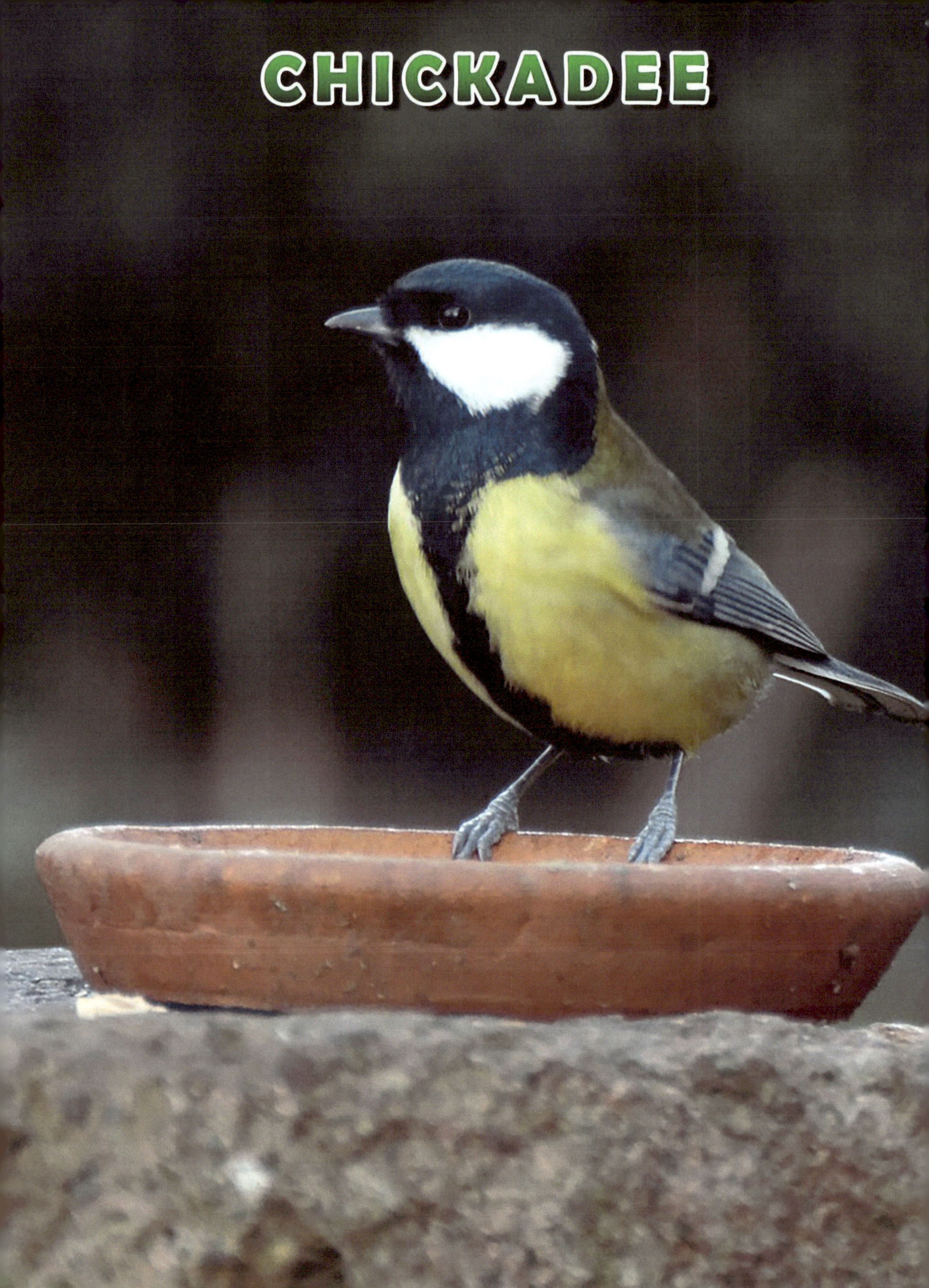

CLARK'S NUTCRACKER

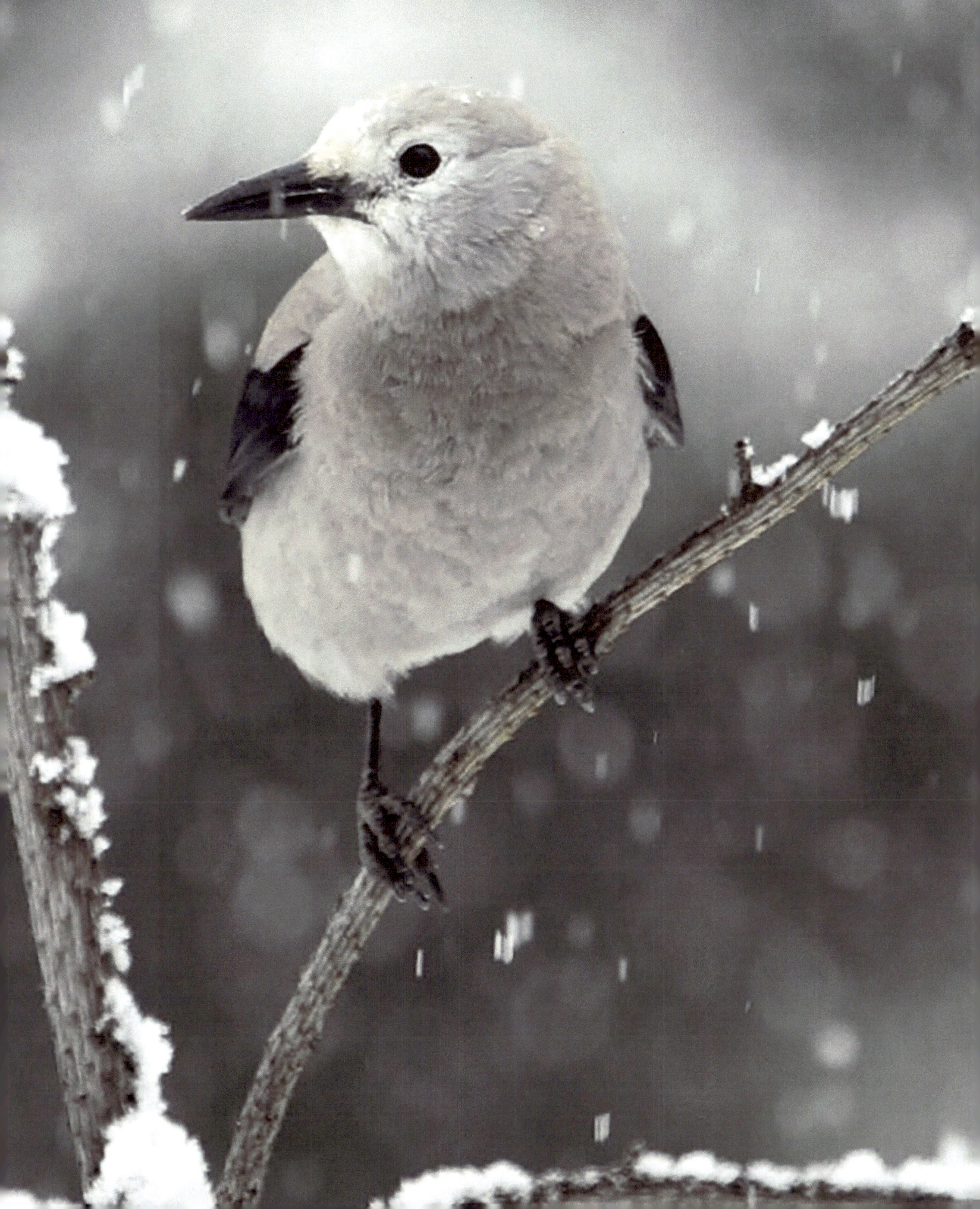

CRESTED BUNTING

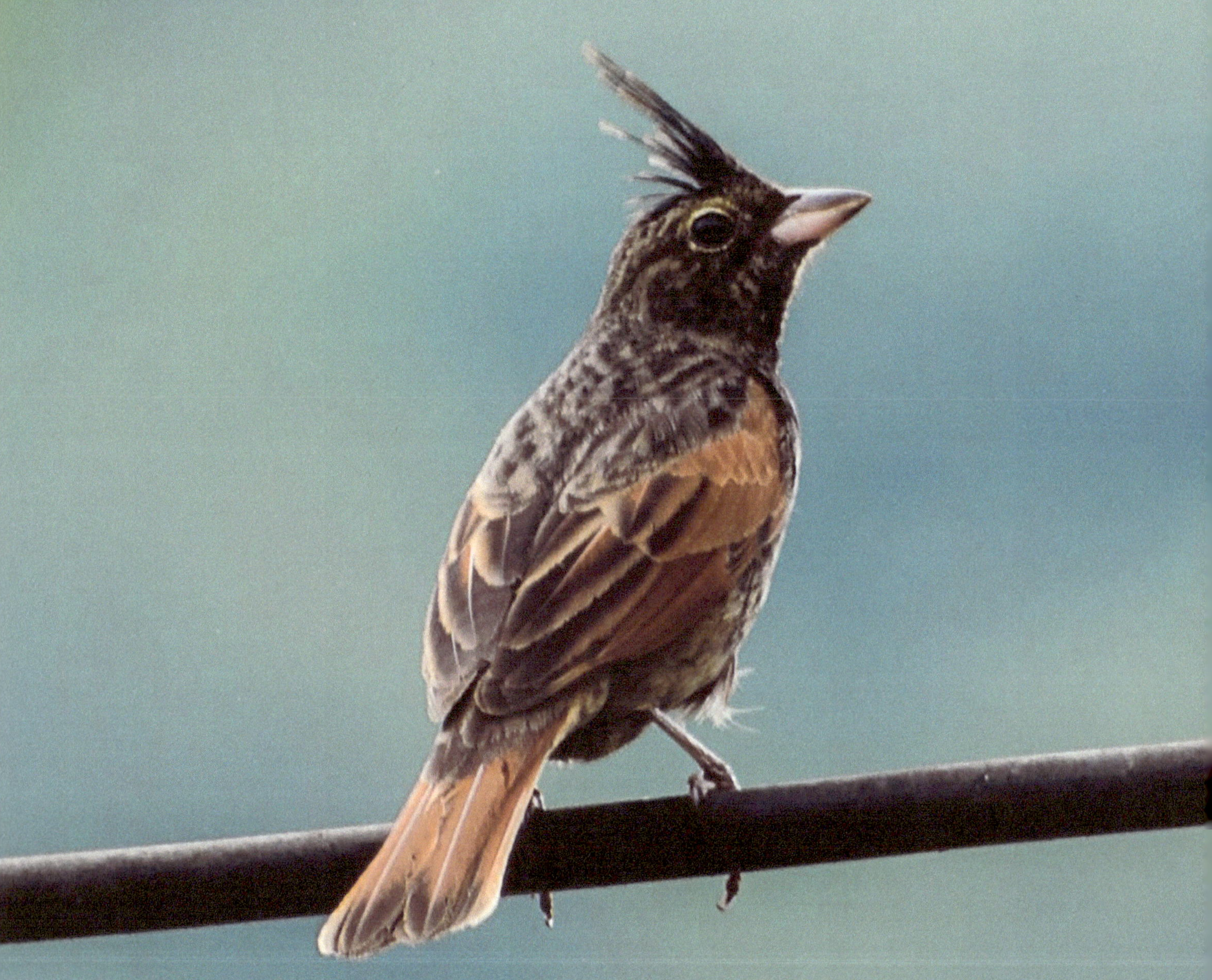

EGRETS (HERONS)

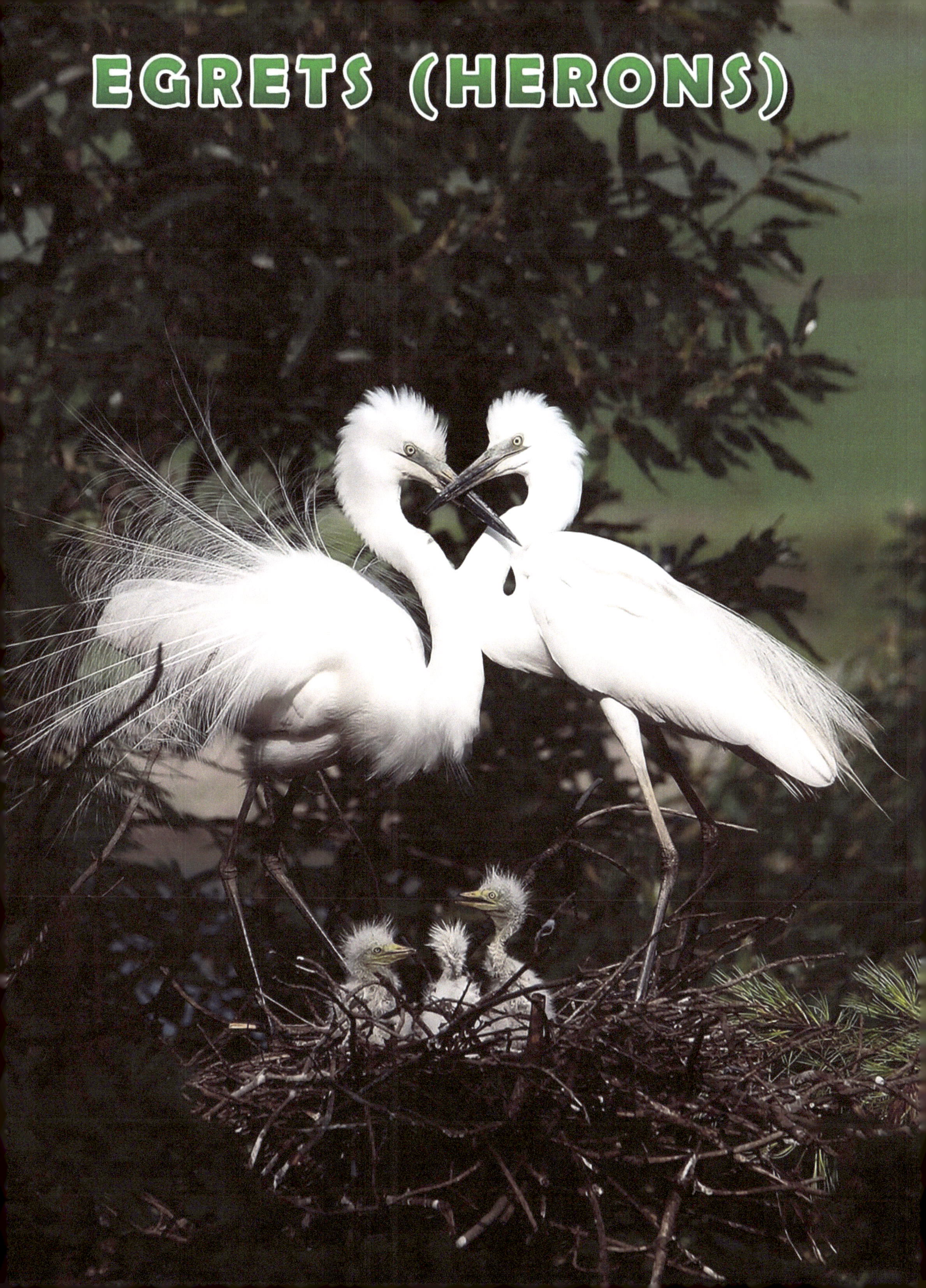

EURASIAN JAY

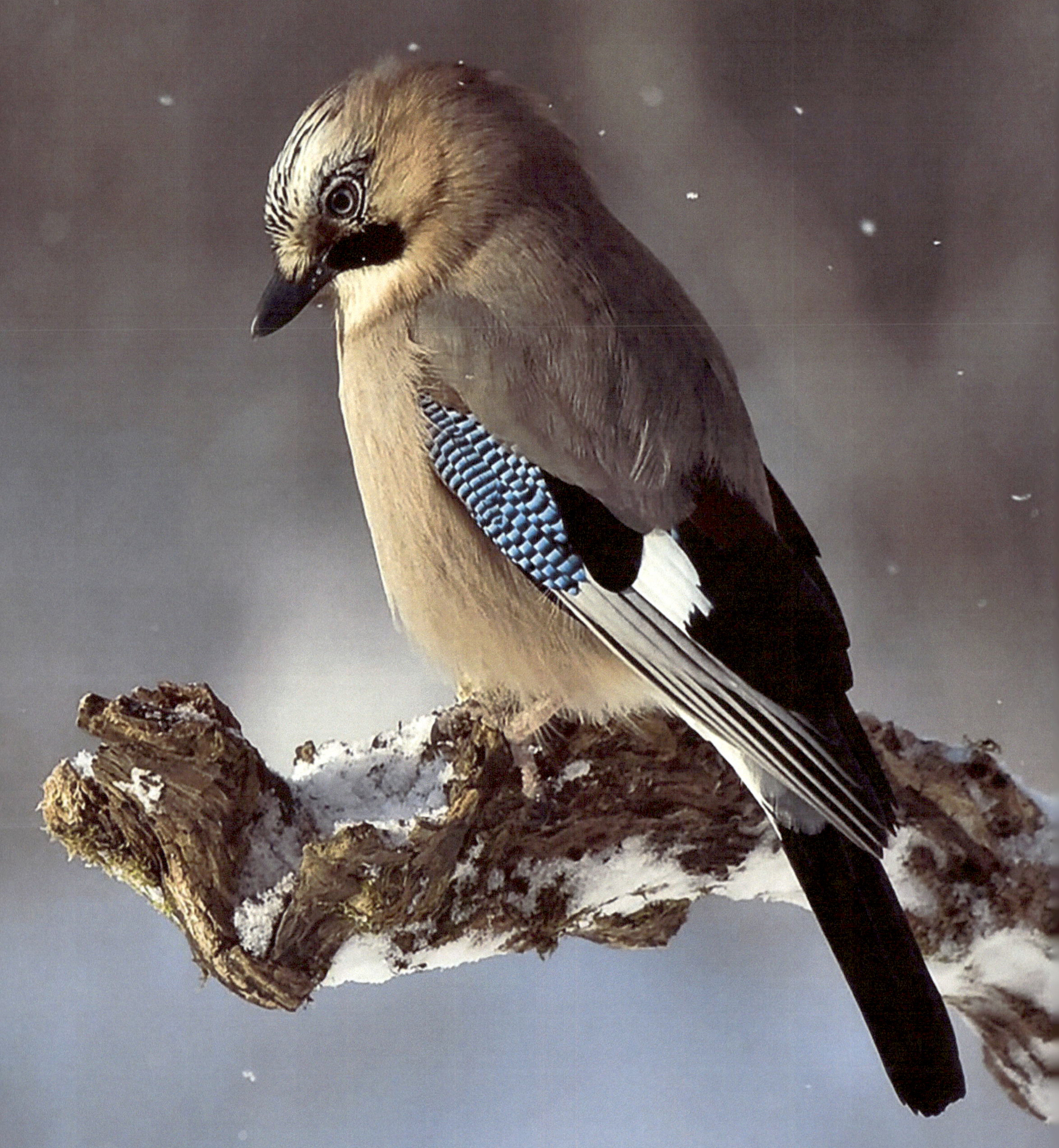

EUROPEAN GOLDFINCH

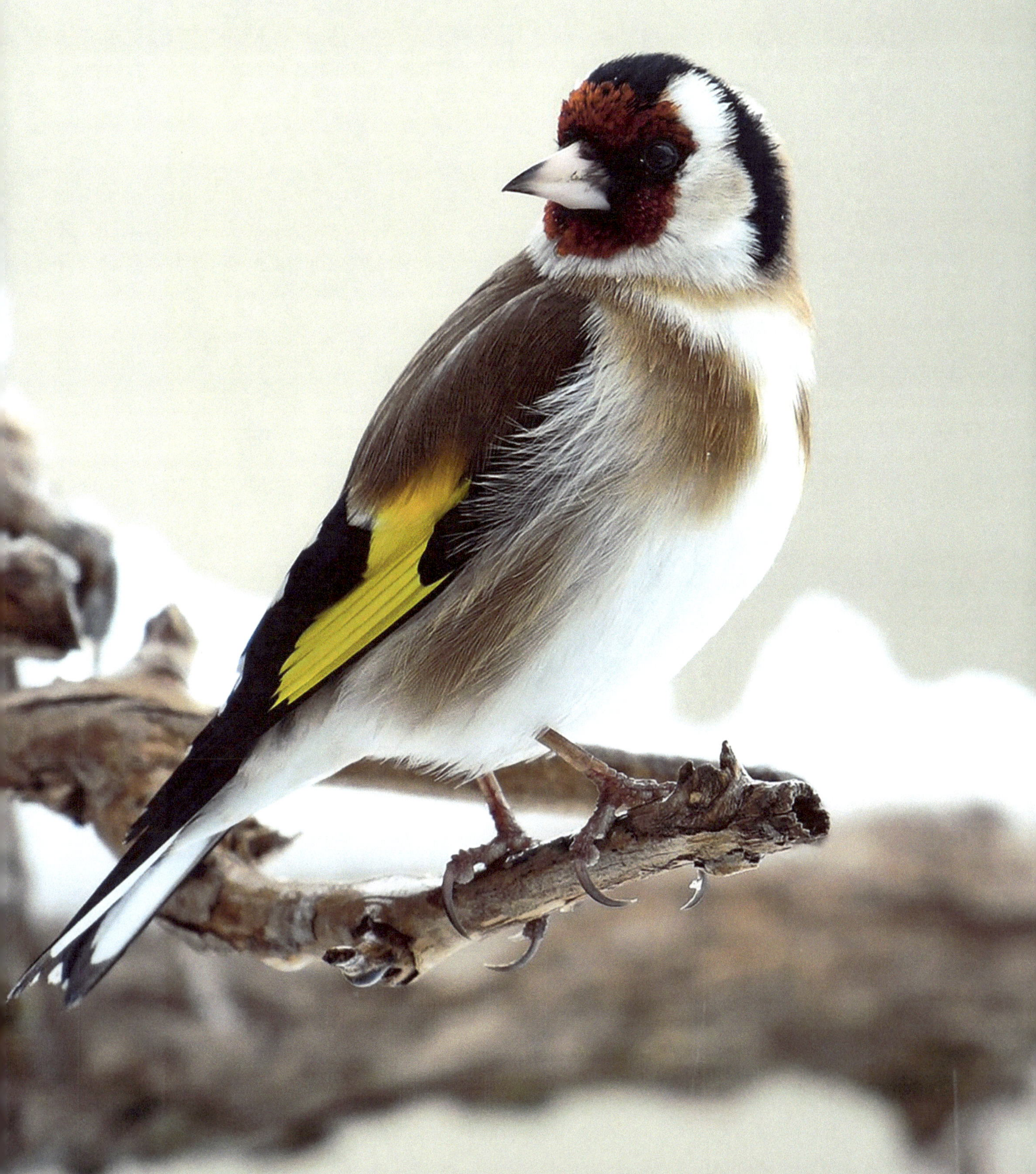

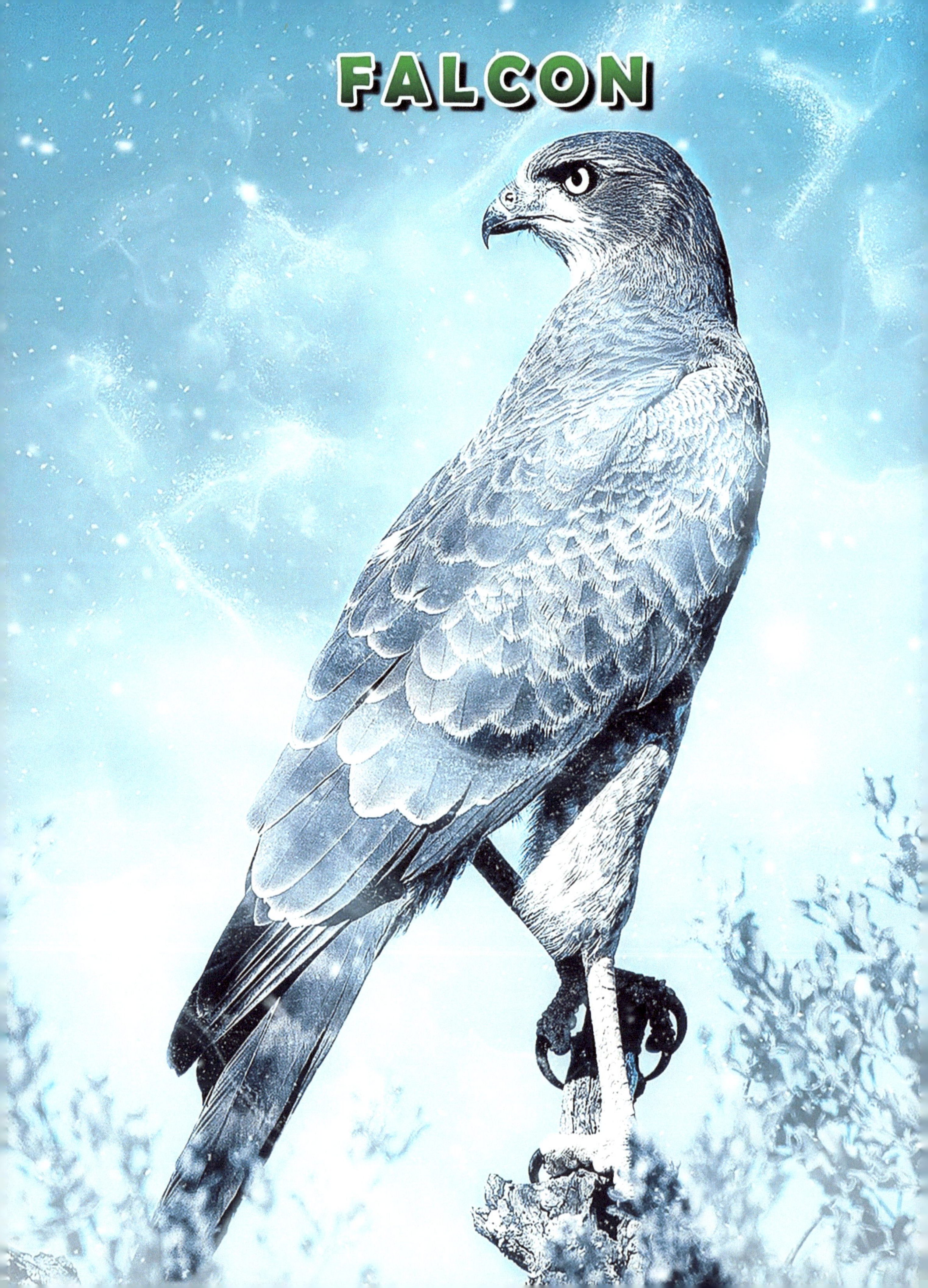

FALCON

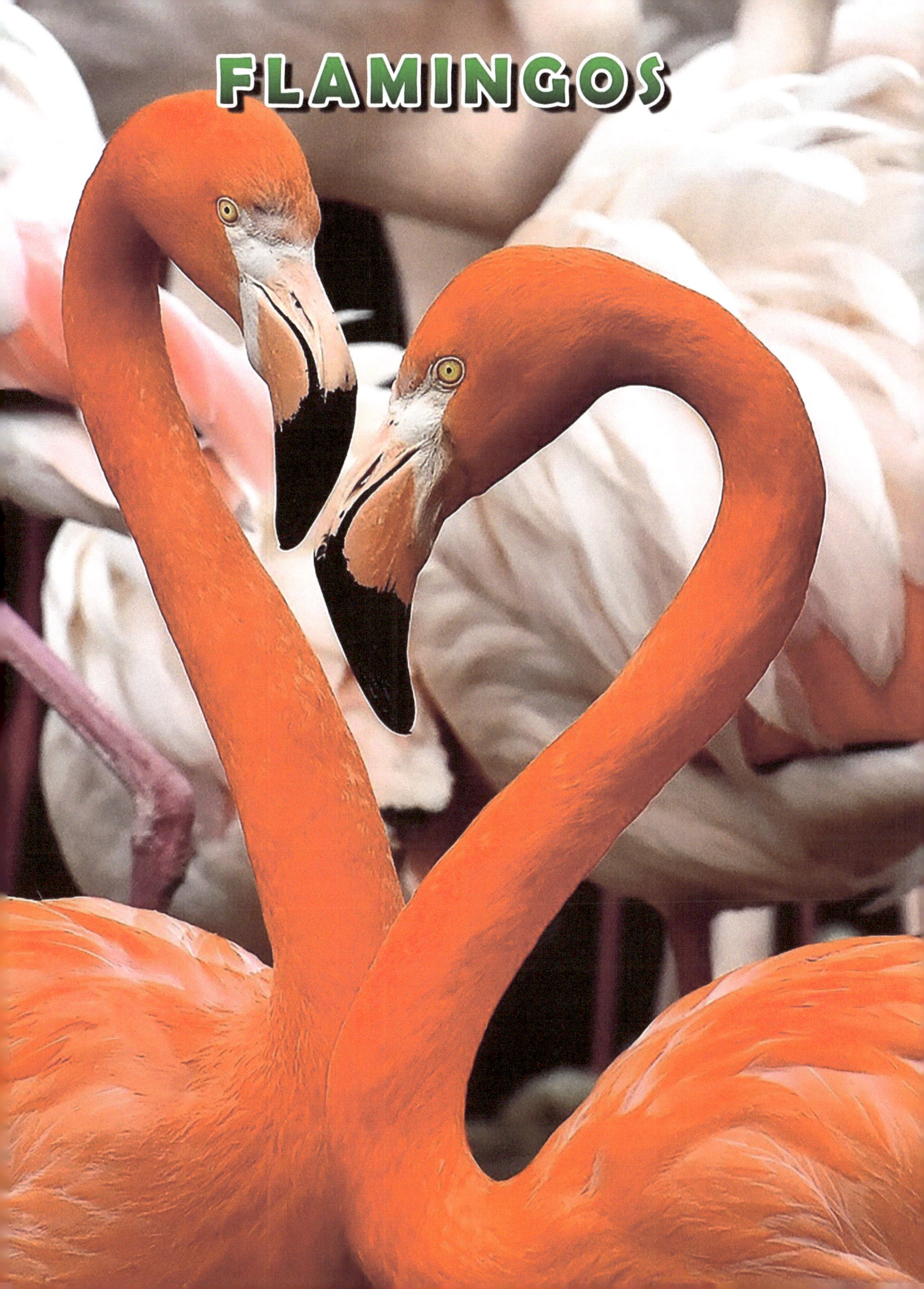
FLAMINGOS

GOULDIAN FINCH

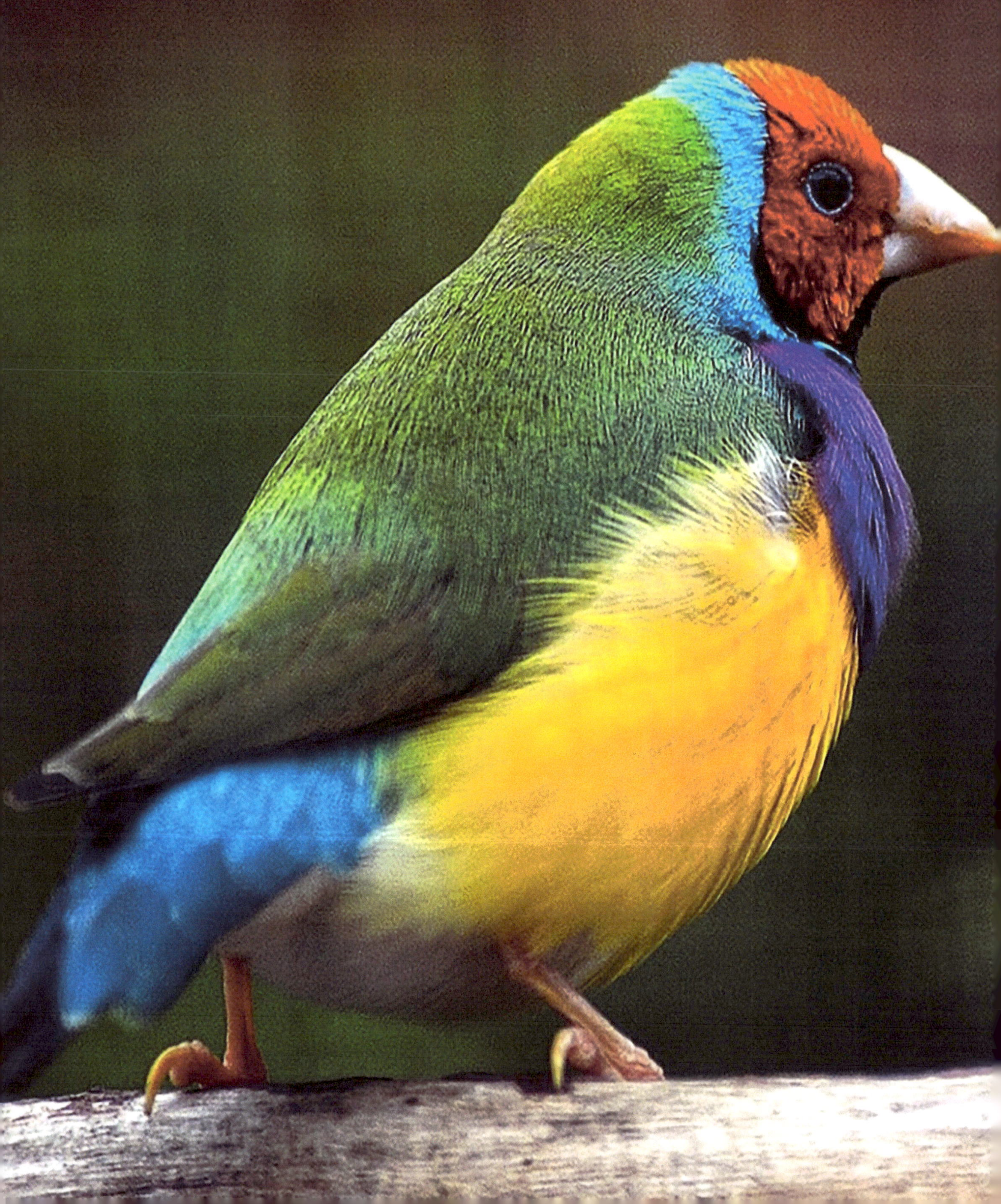

GREATER ROADRUNNER

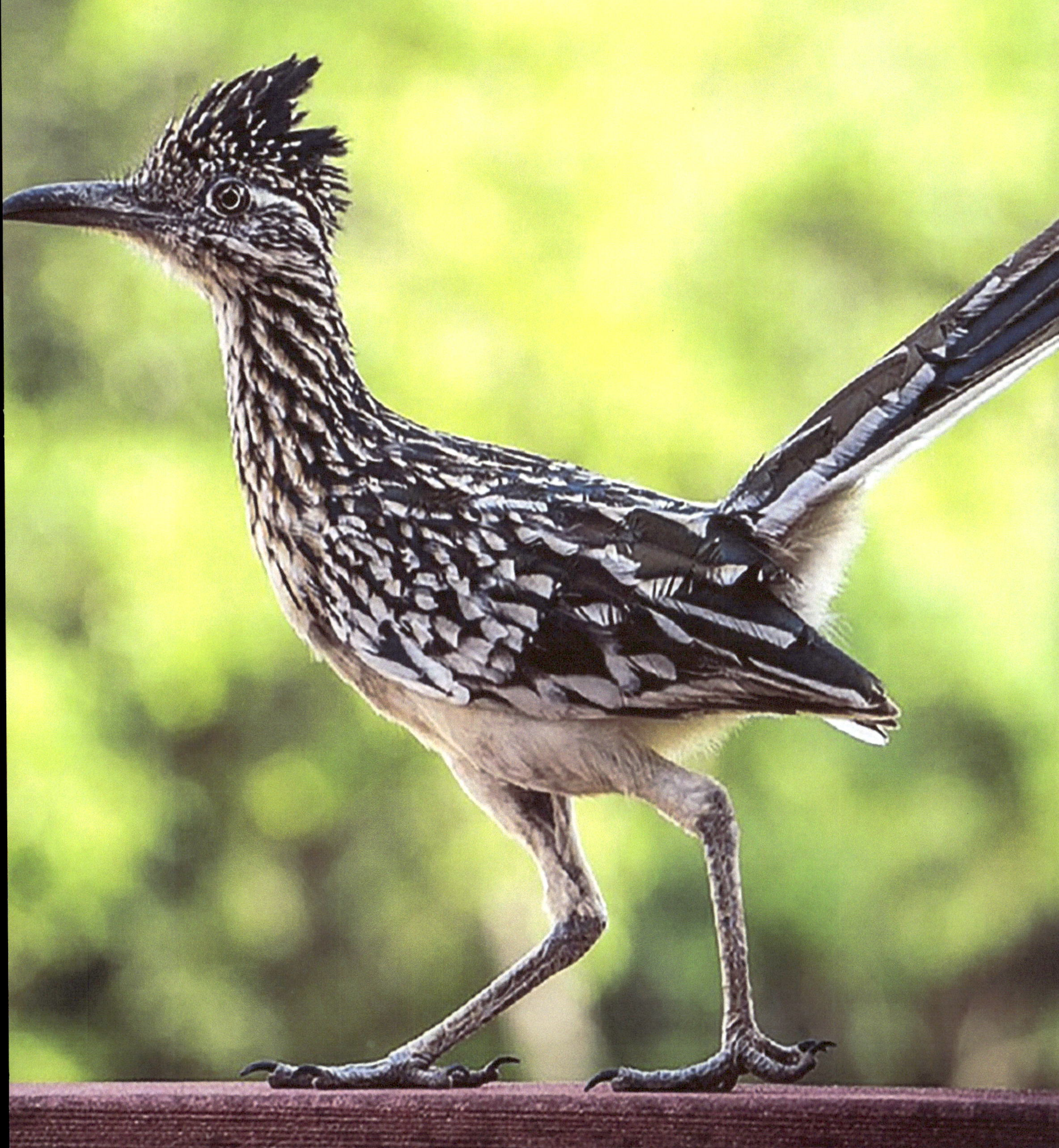

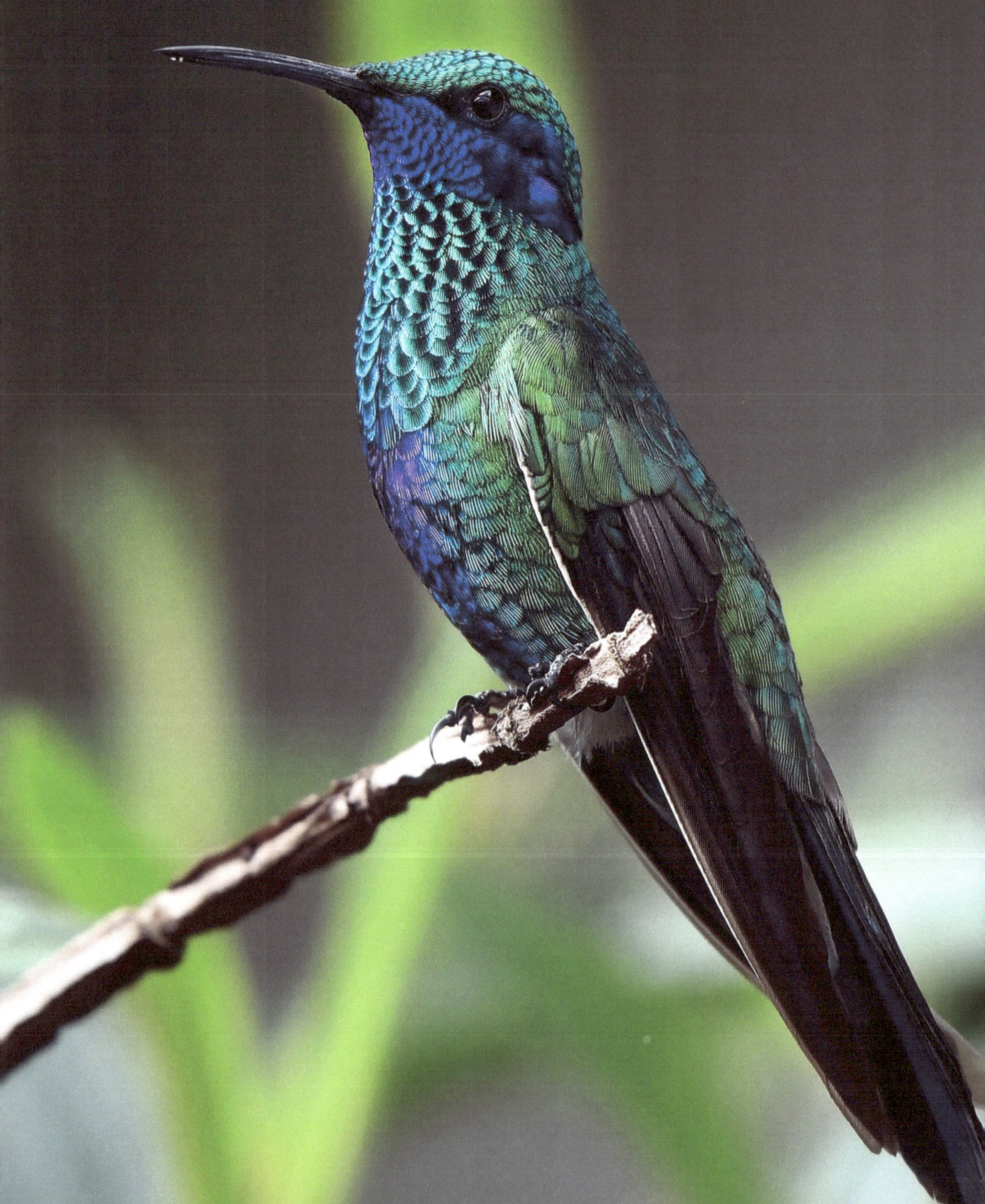

HUMMINGBIRD

HORNBILL

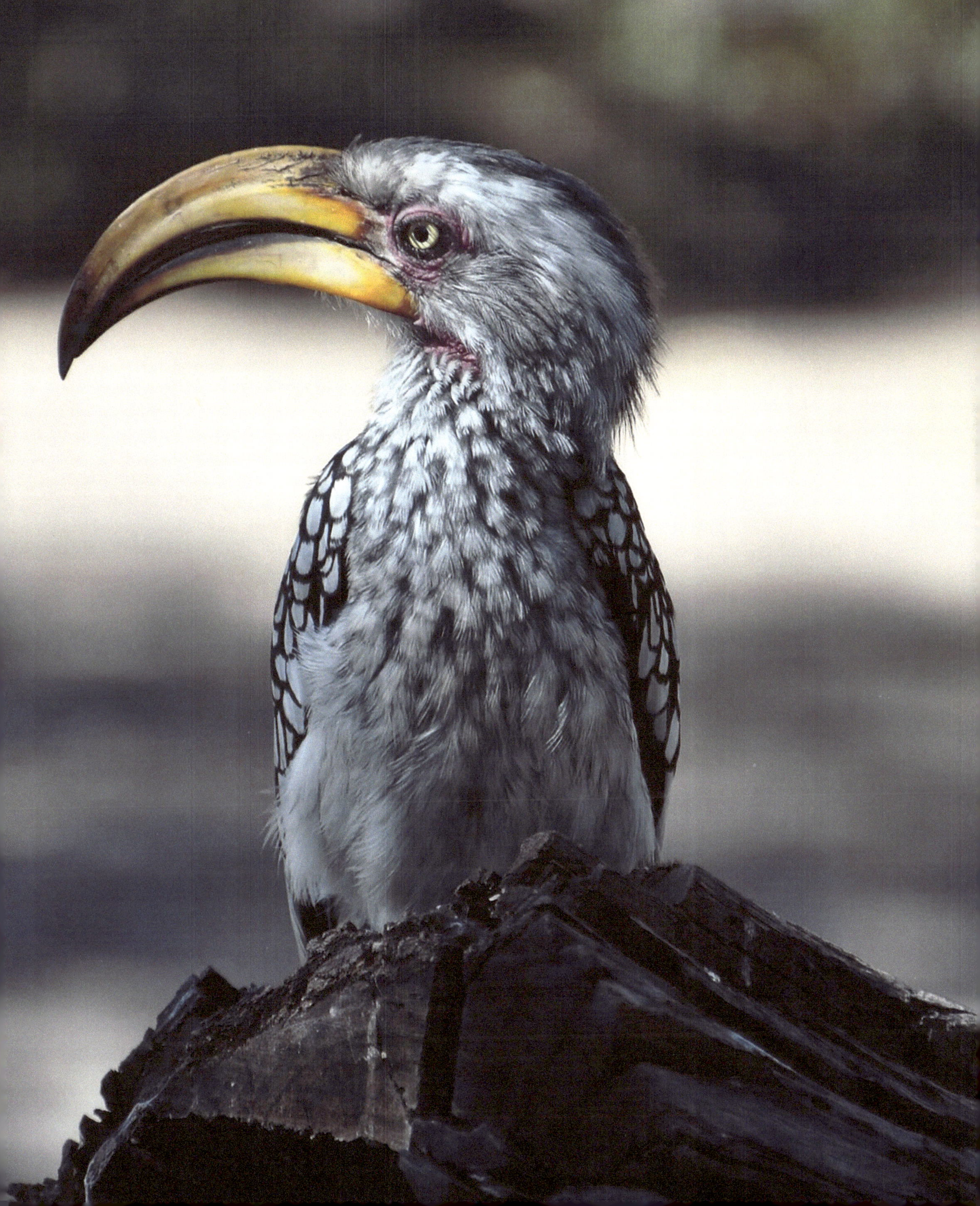

KINGFISHER

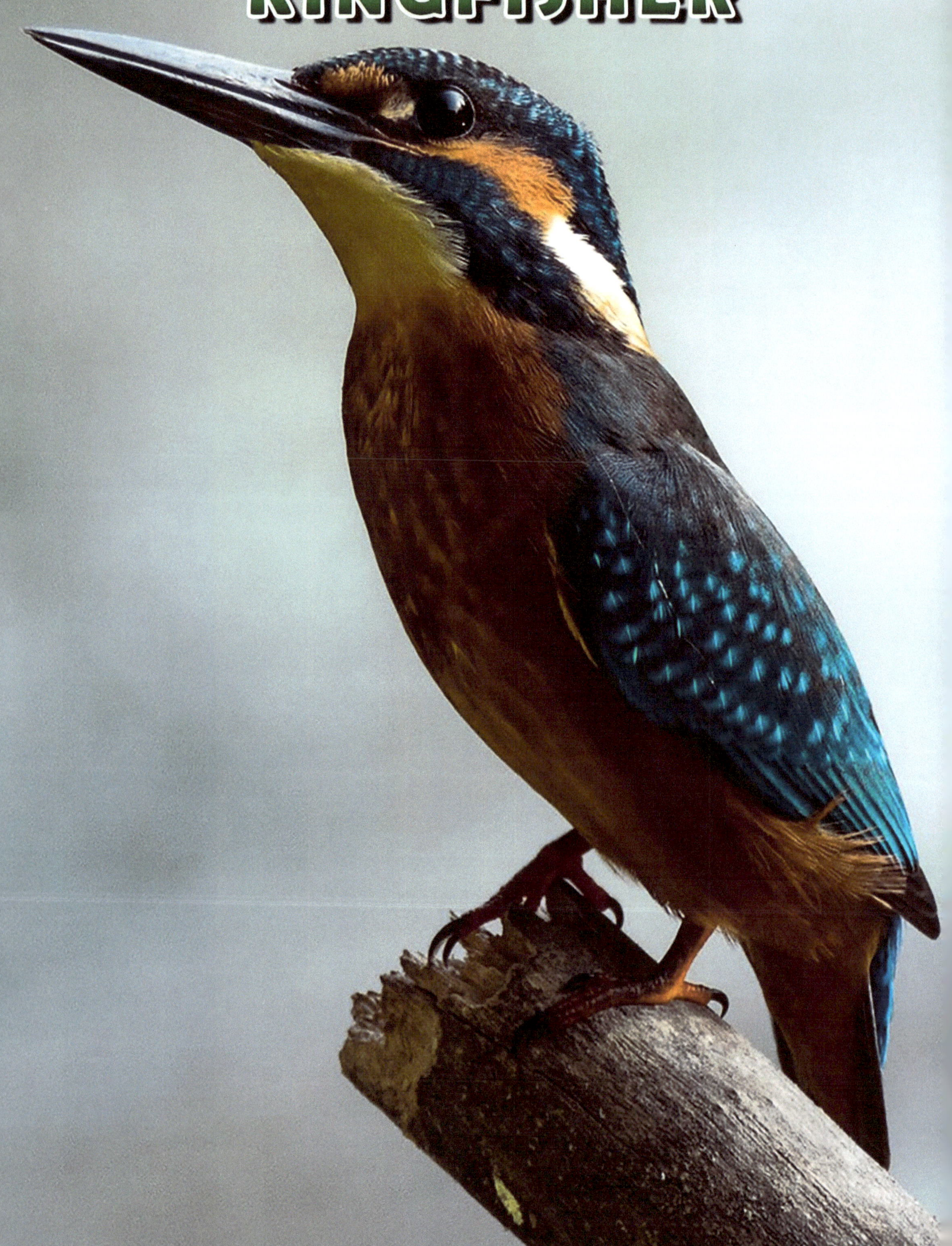

LARK

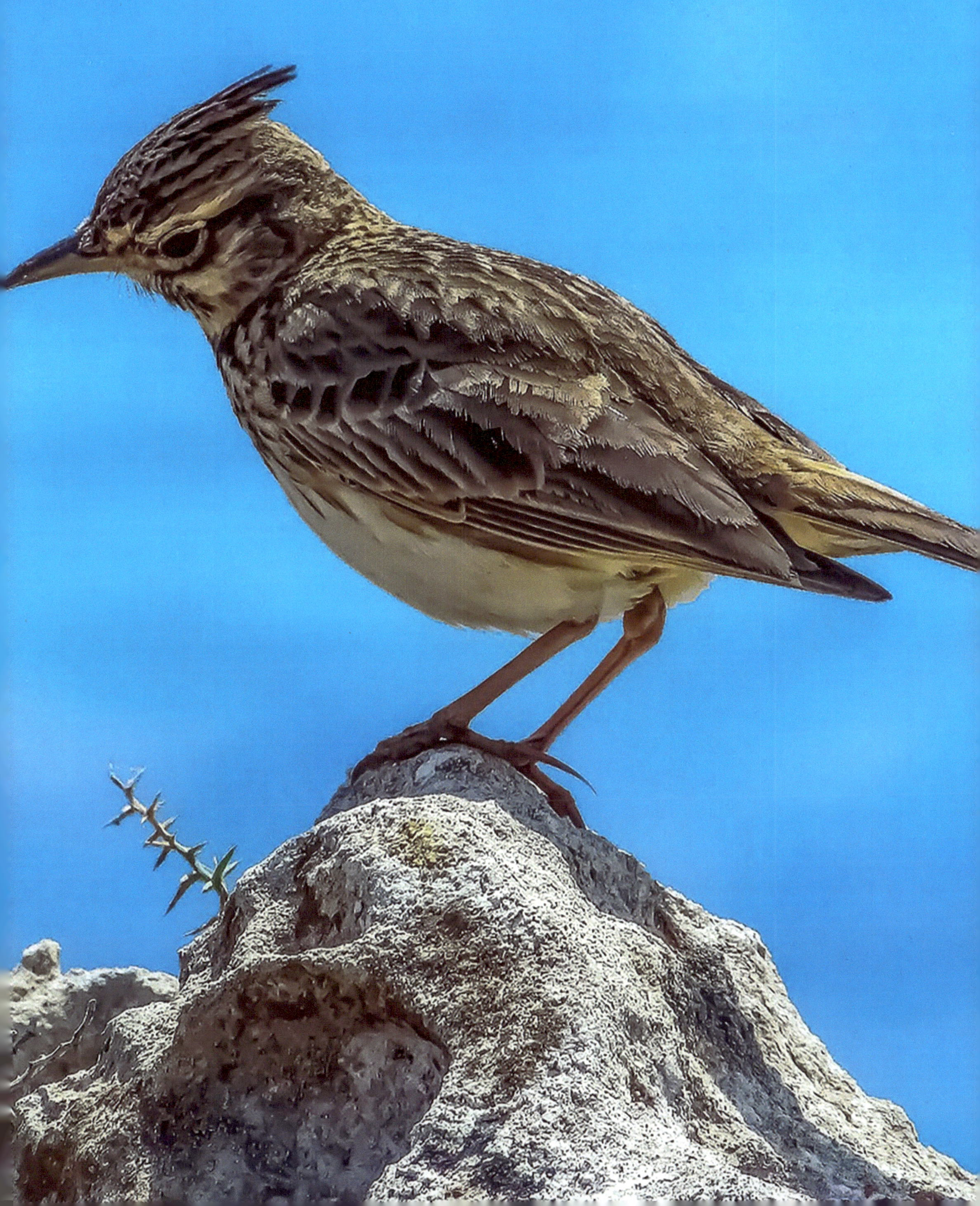

MAGPIE

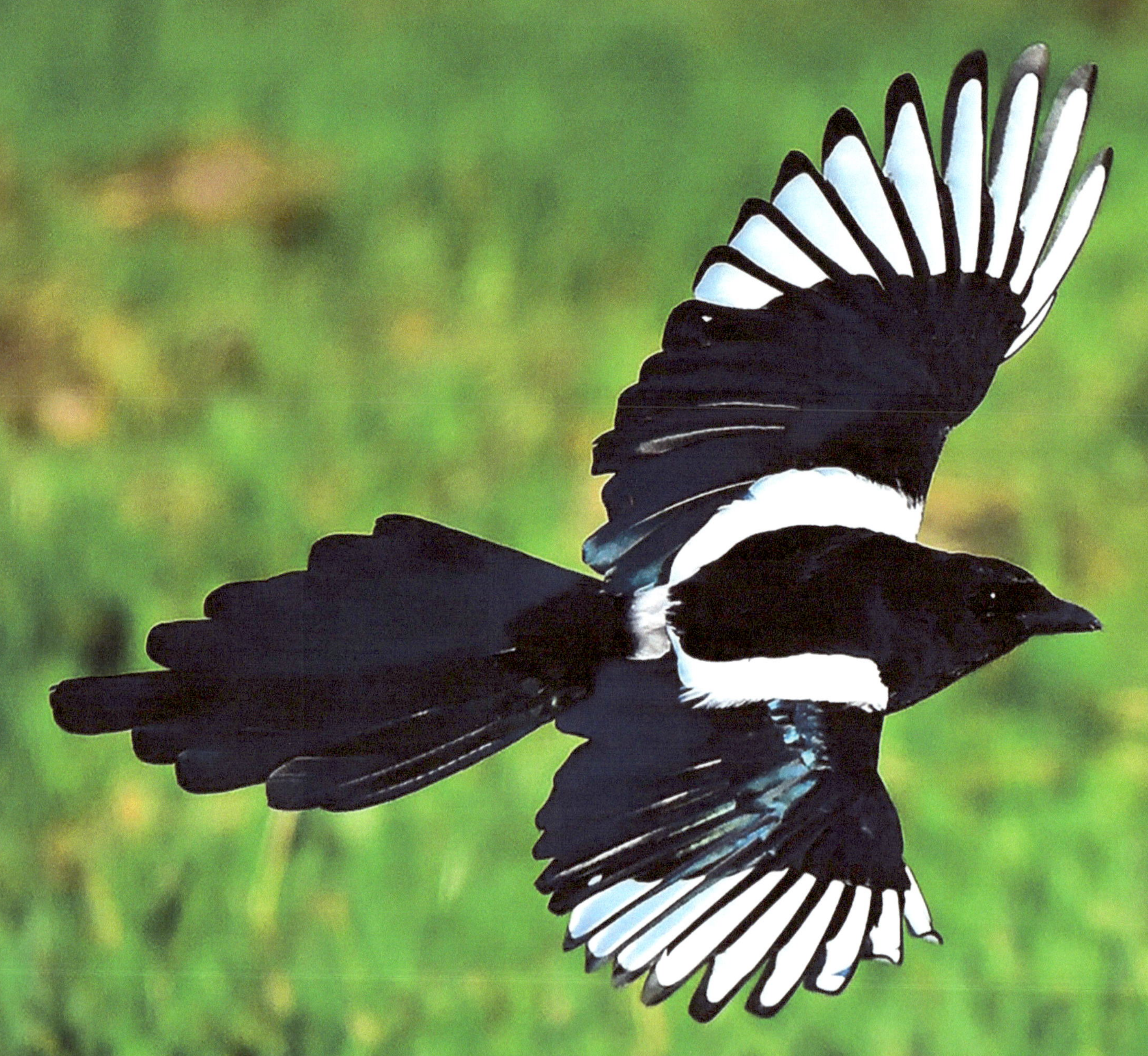

MASKED LAPWING

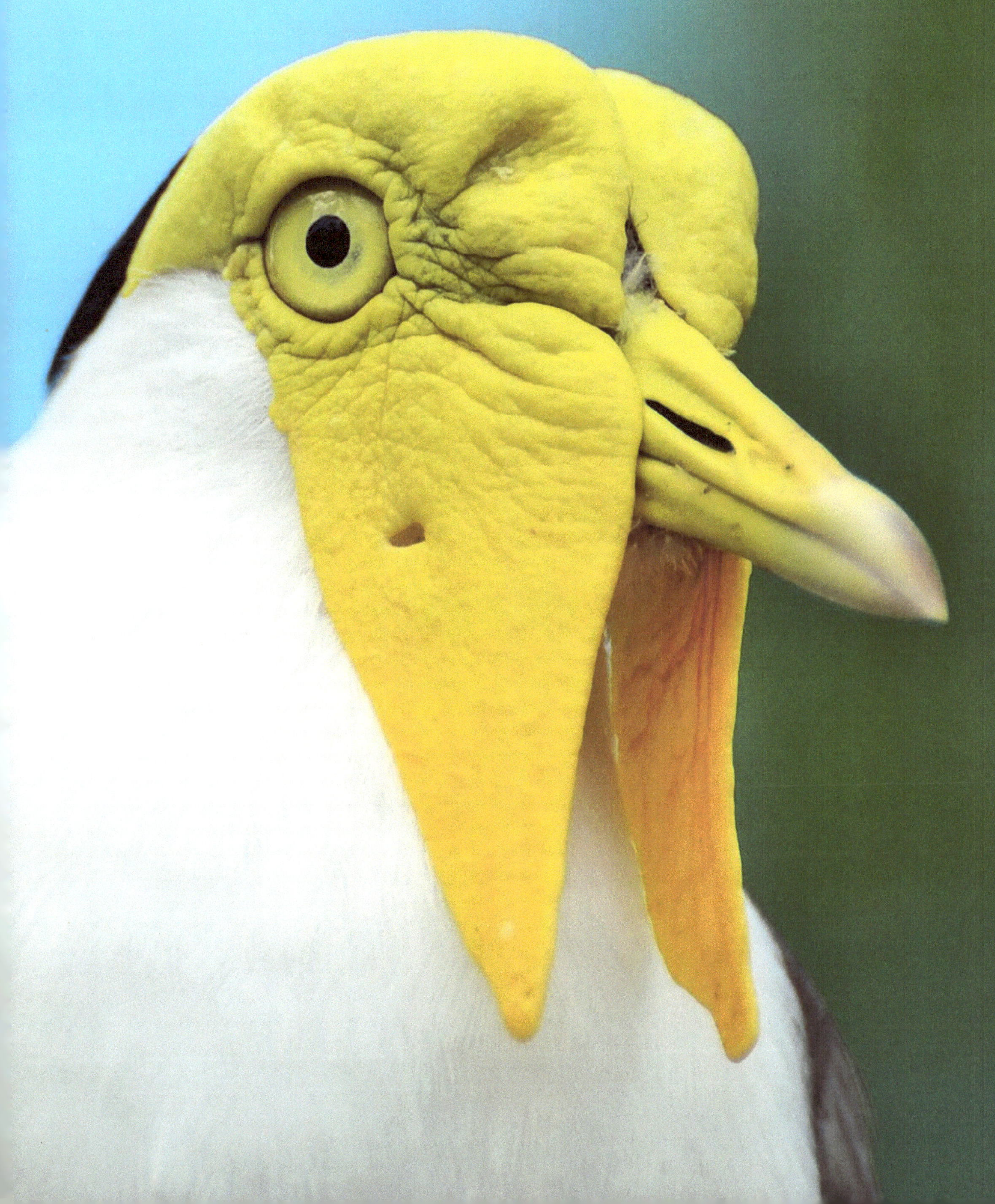

COMMON MERGANSER

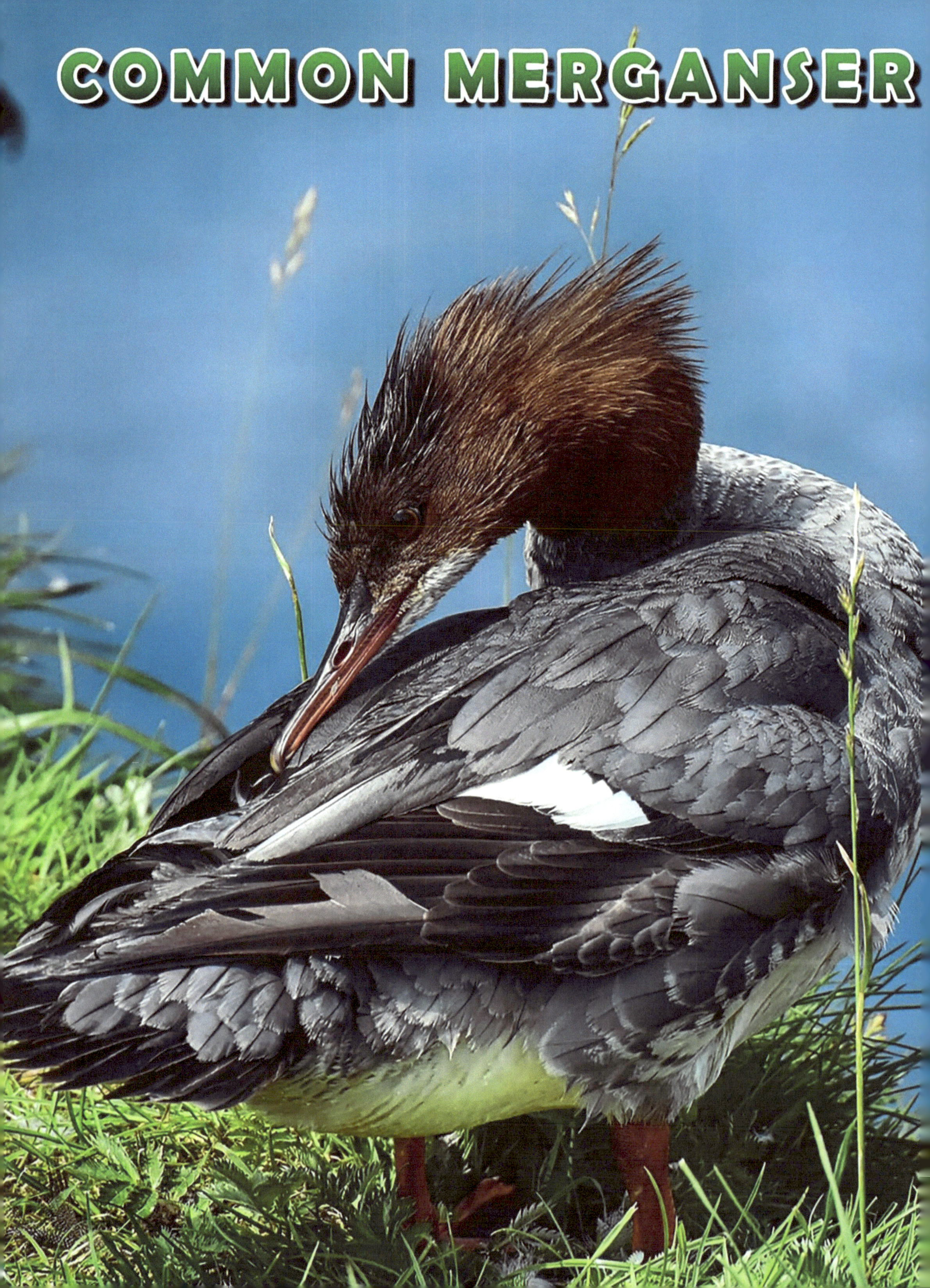

BARN OWL

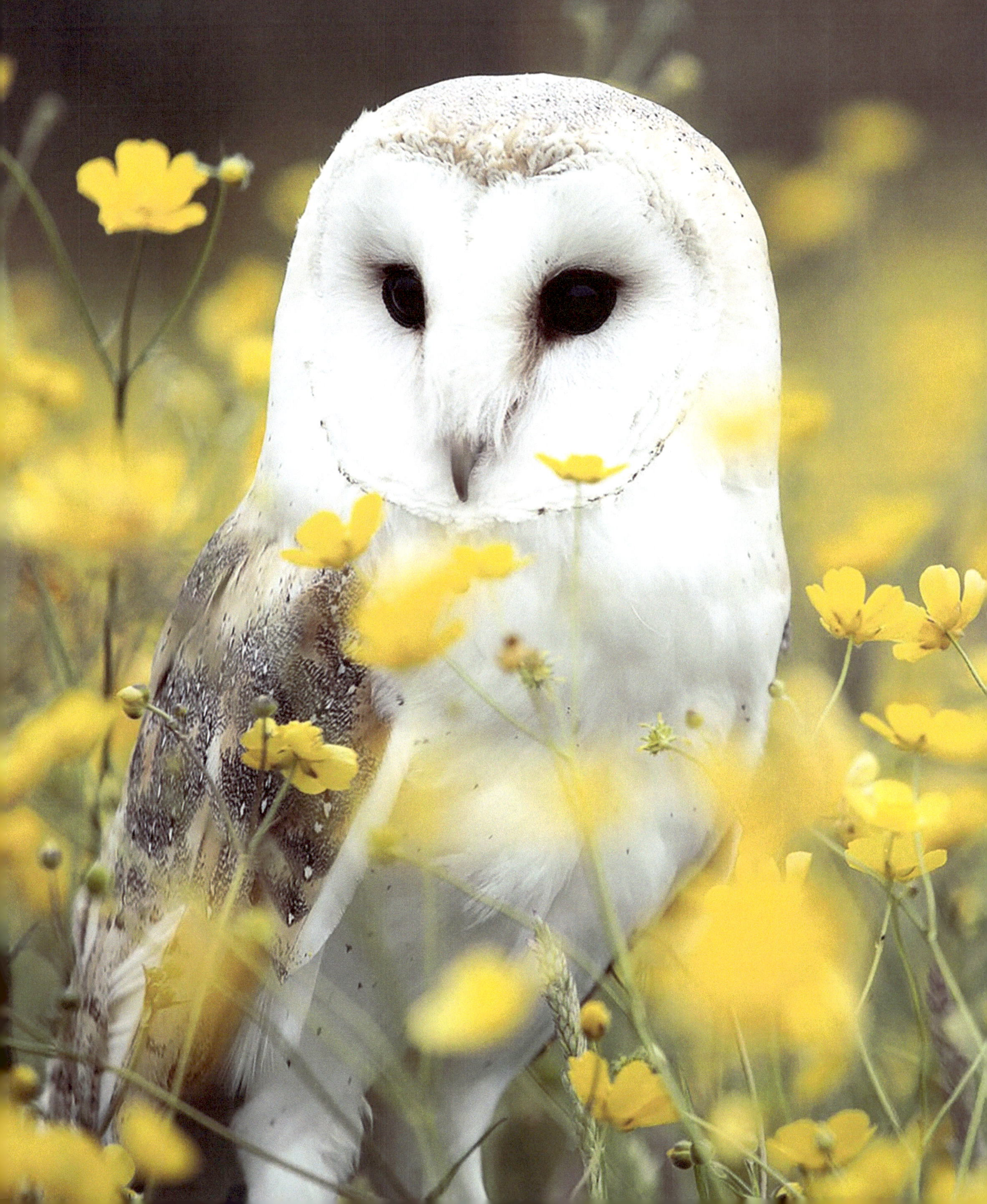

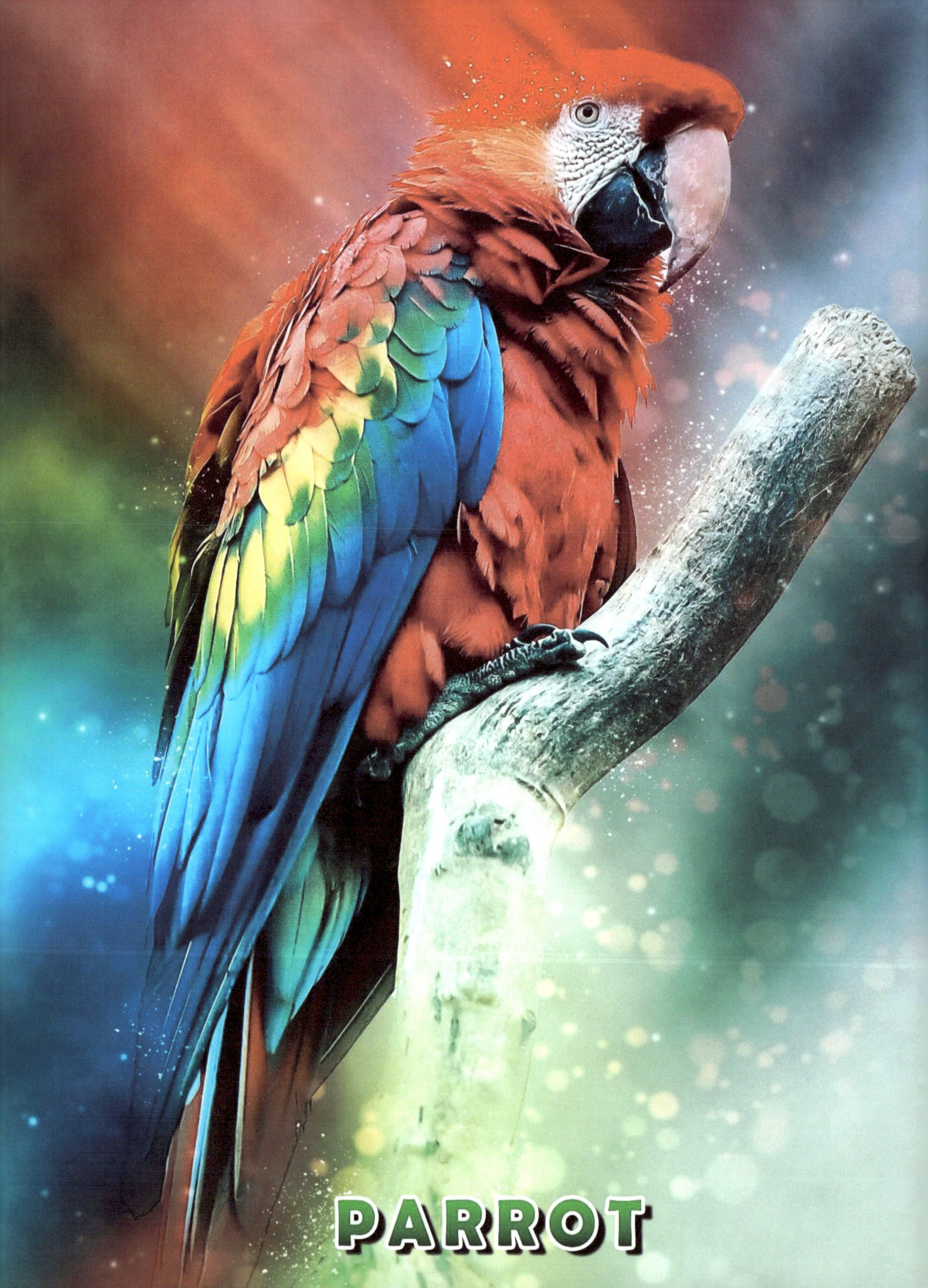

PARROT

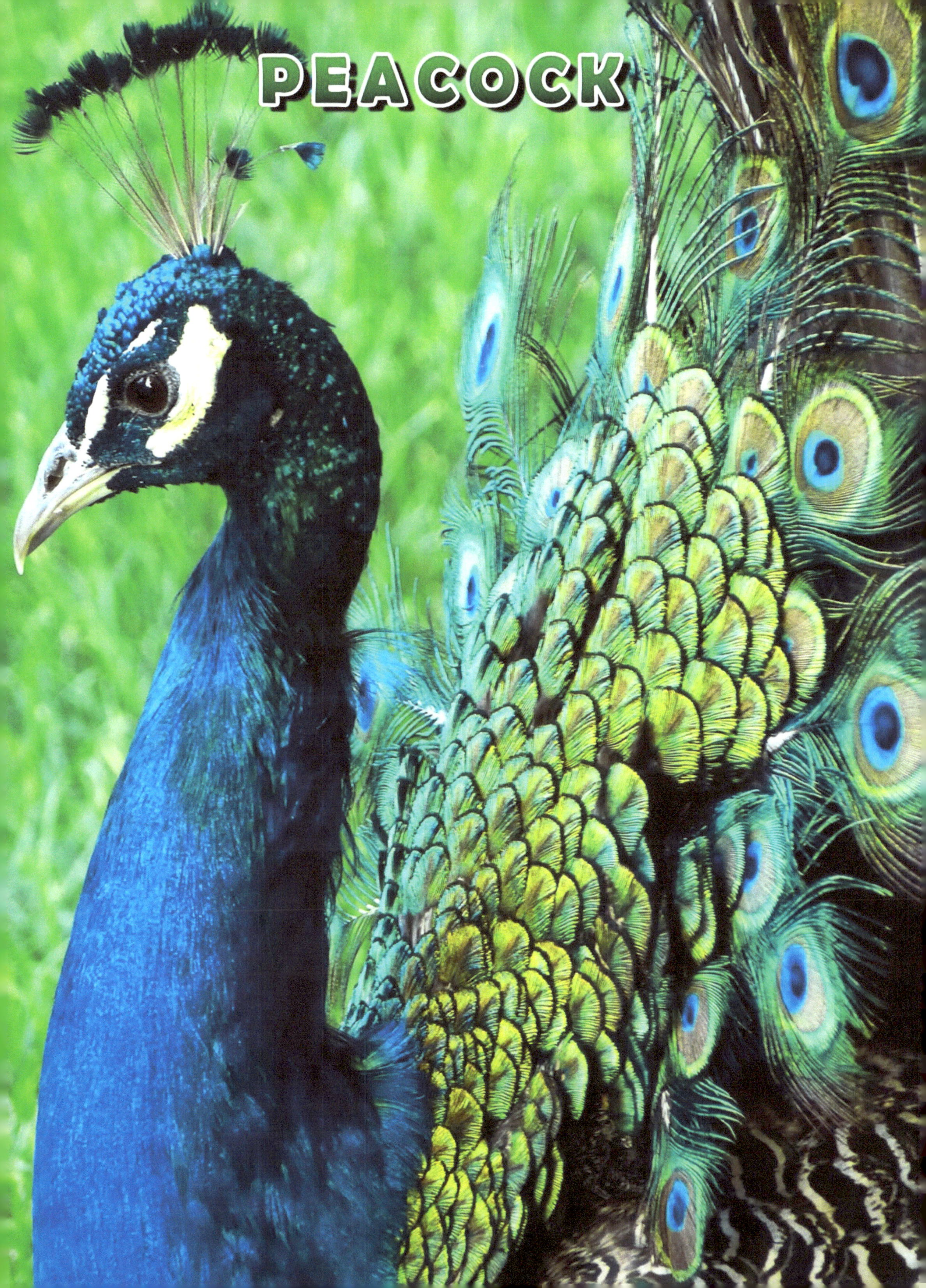
PEACOCK

PELICAN

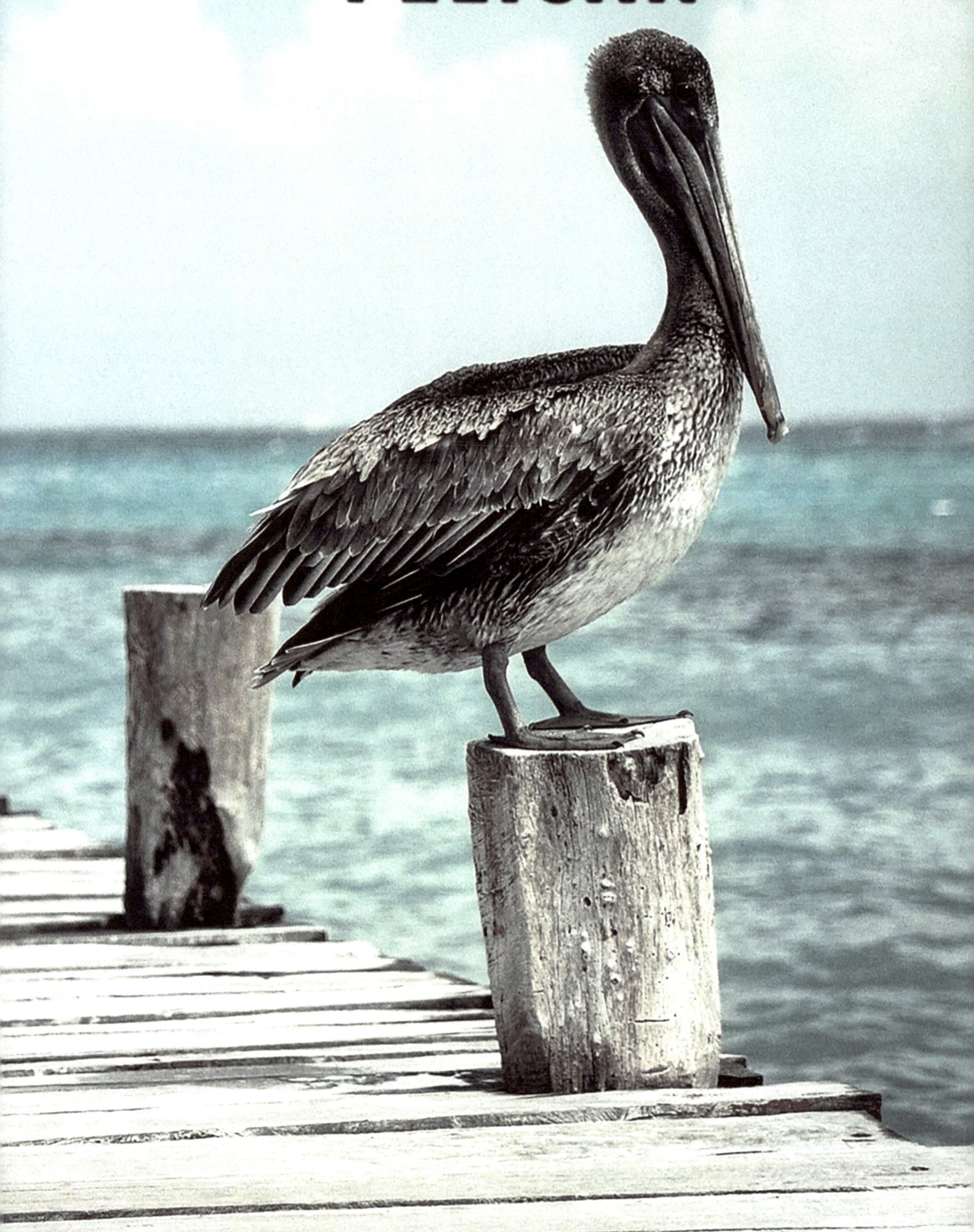

EMPEROR PENGUINS

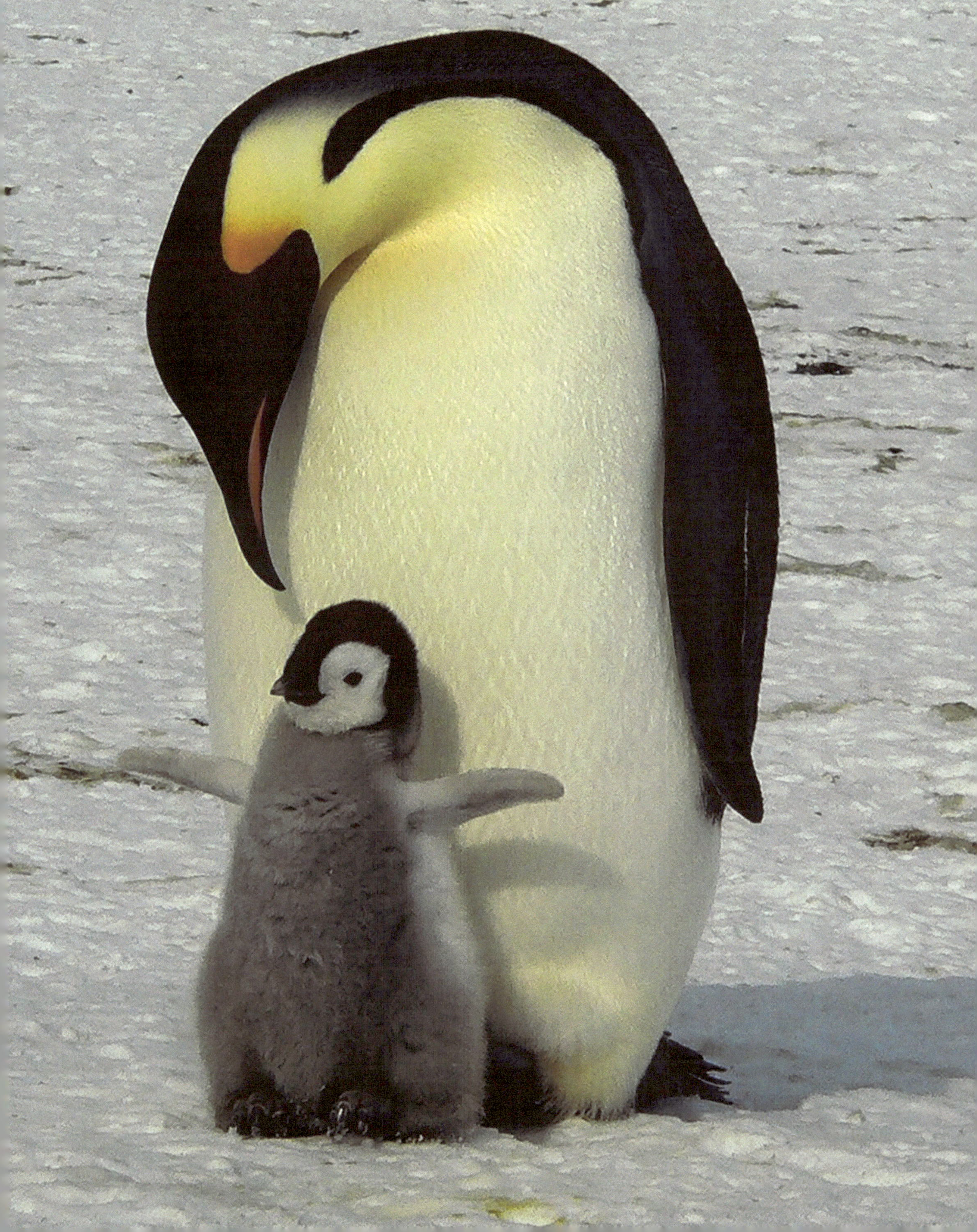

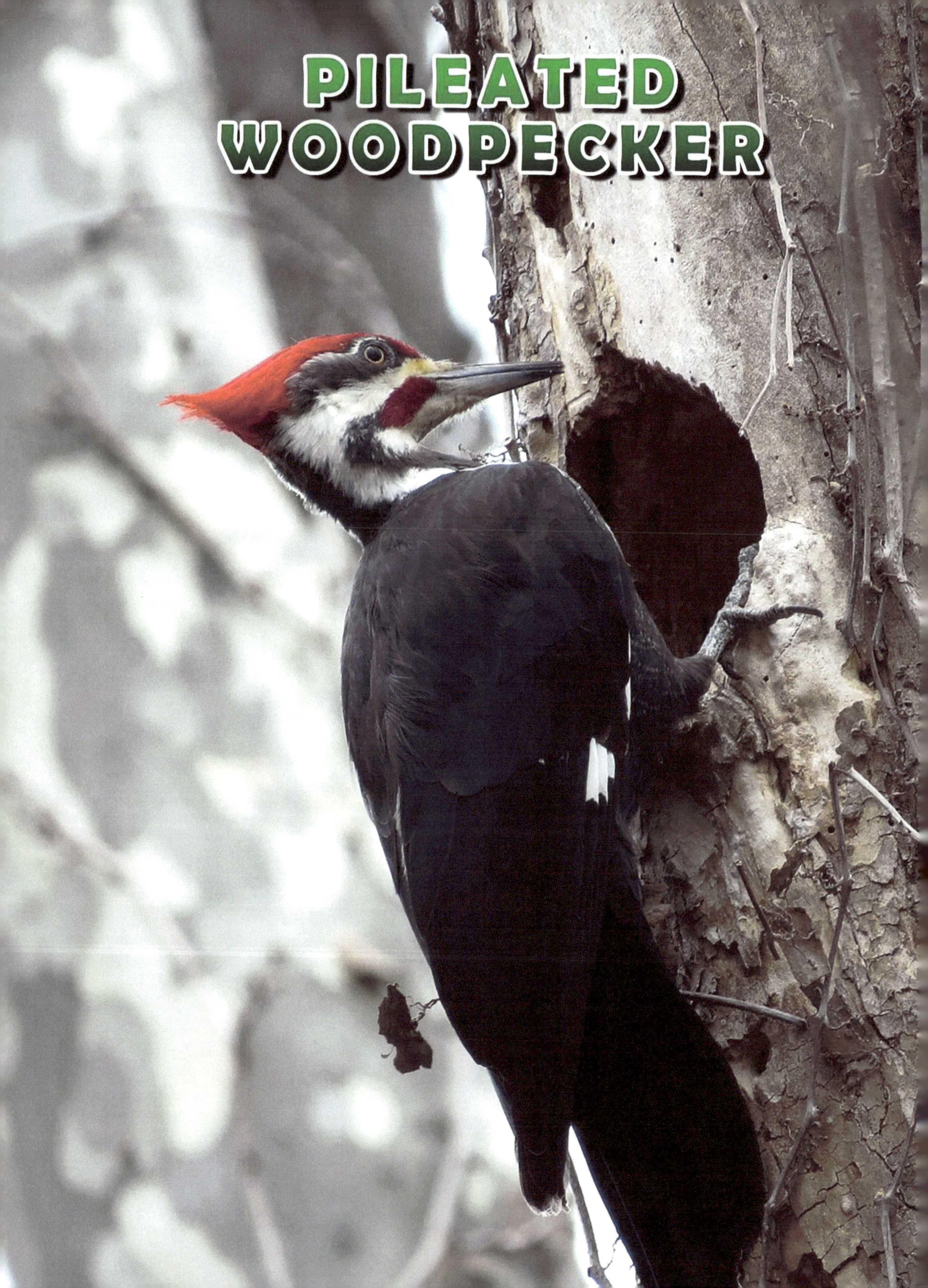
PILEATED
WOODPECKER

RAINBOW LORIKEET

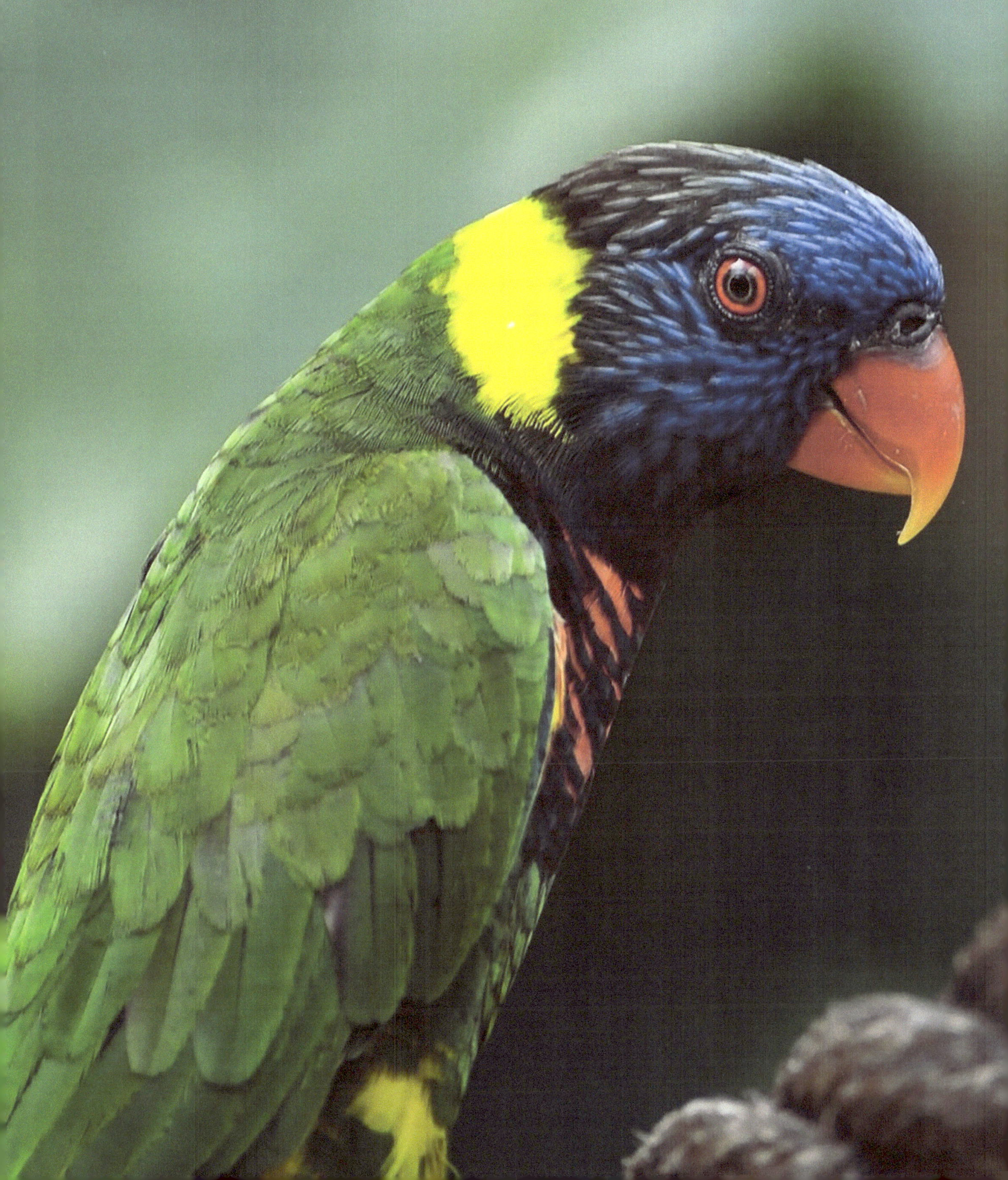

AMERICAN ROBIN

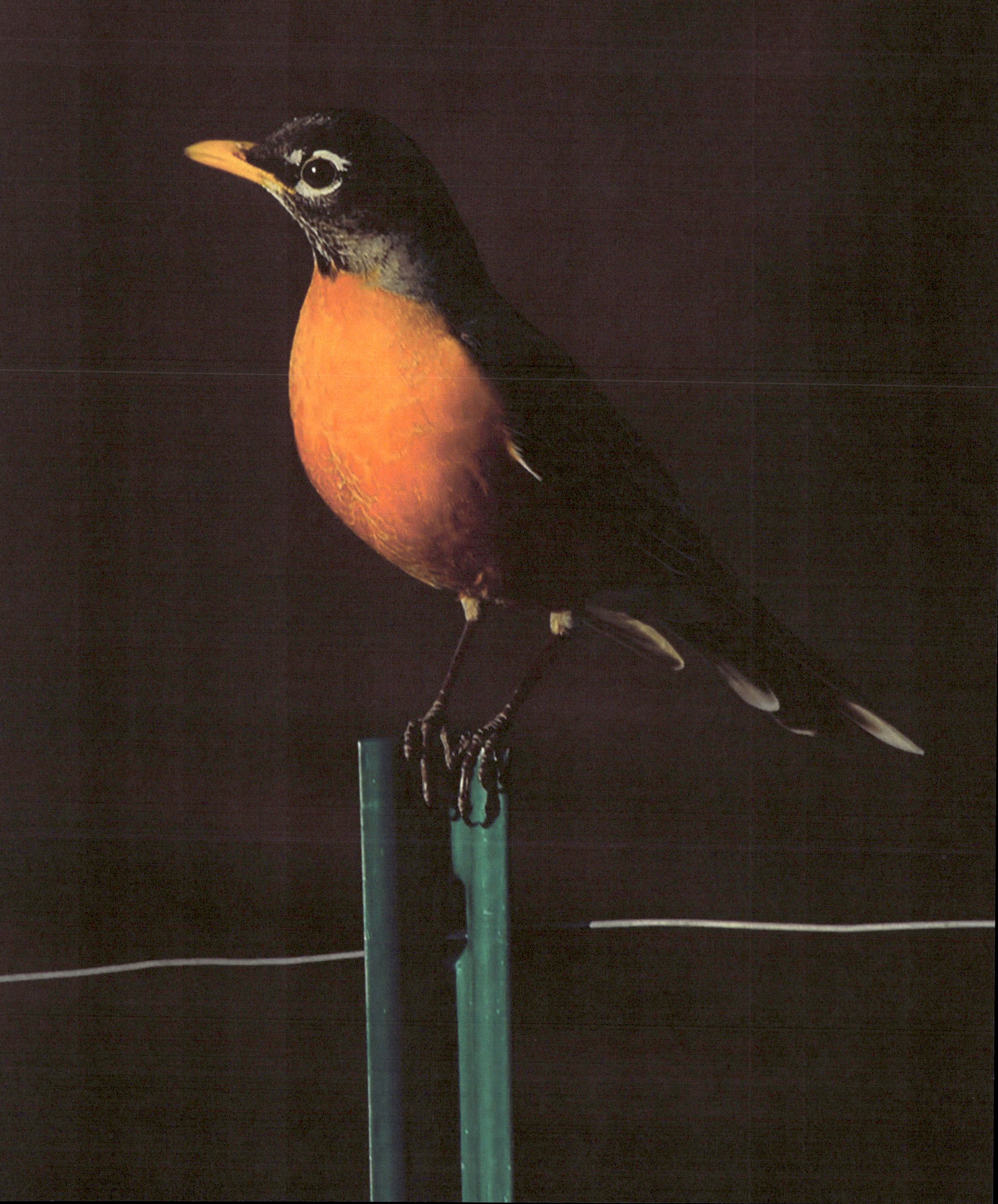

SEAGULL

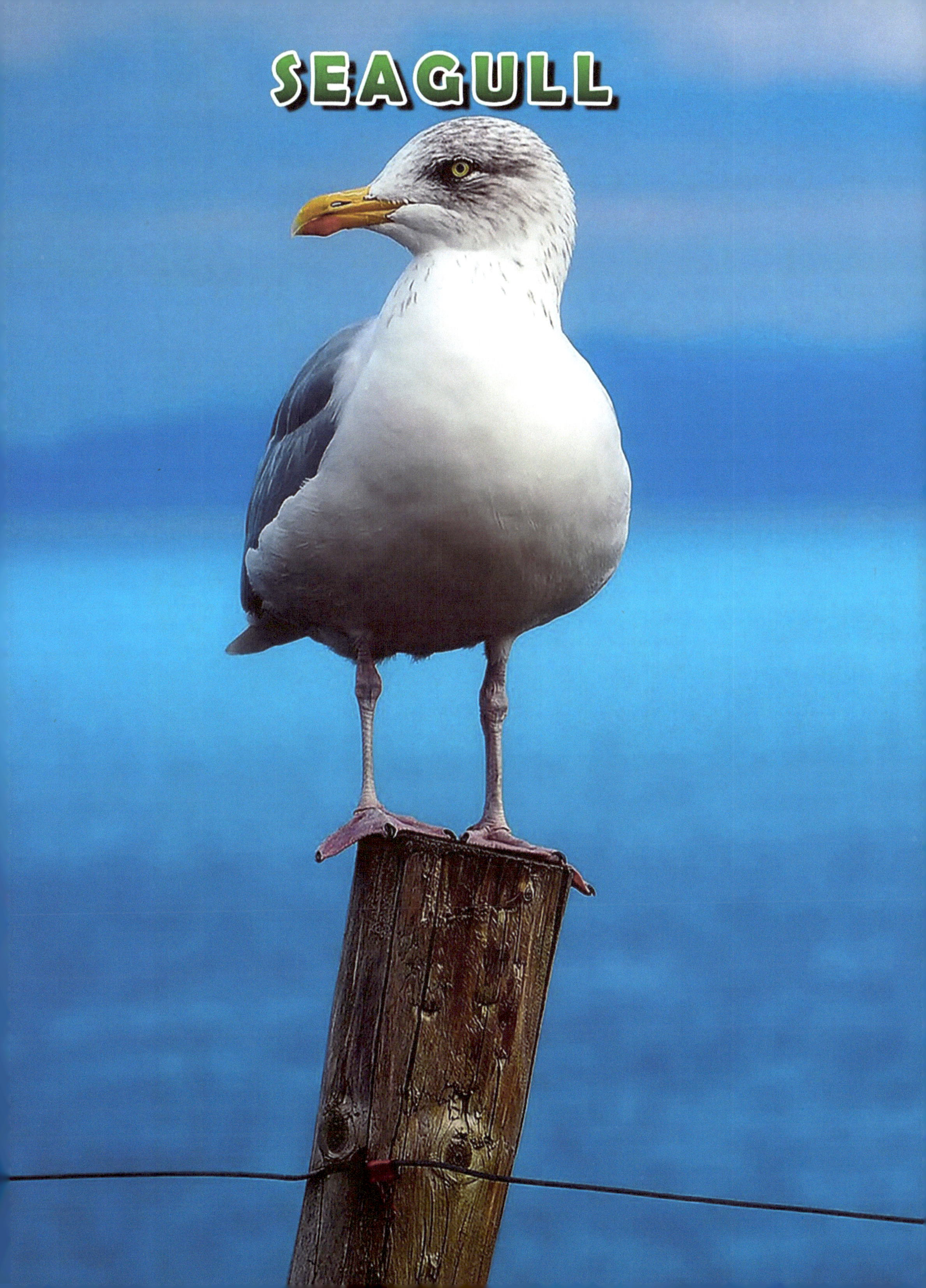

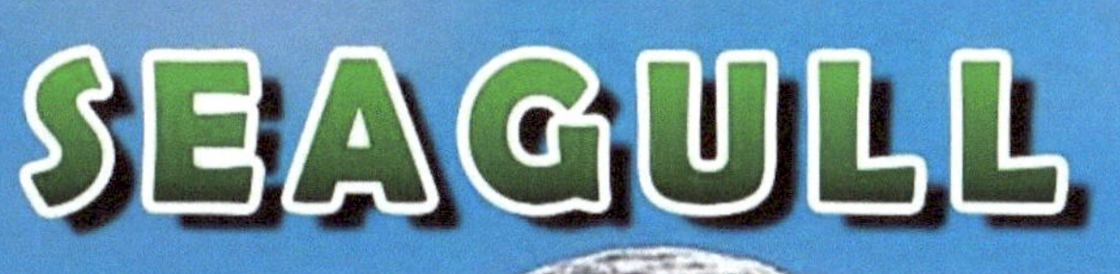

SPARROW

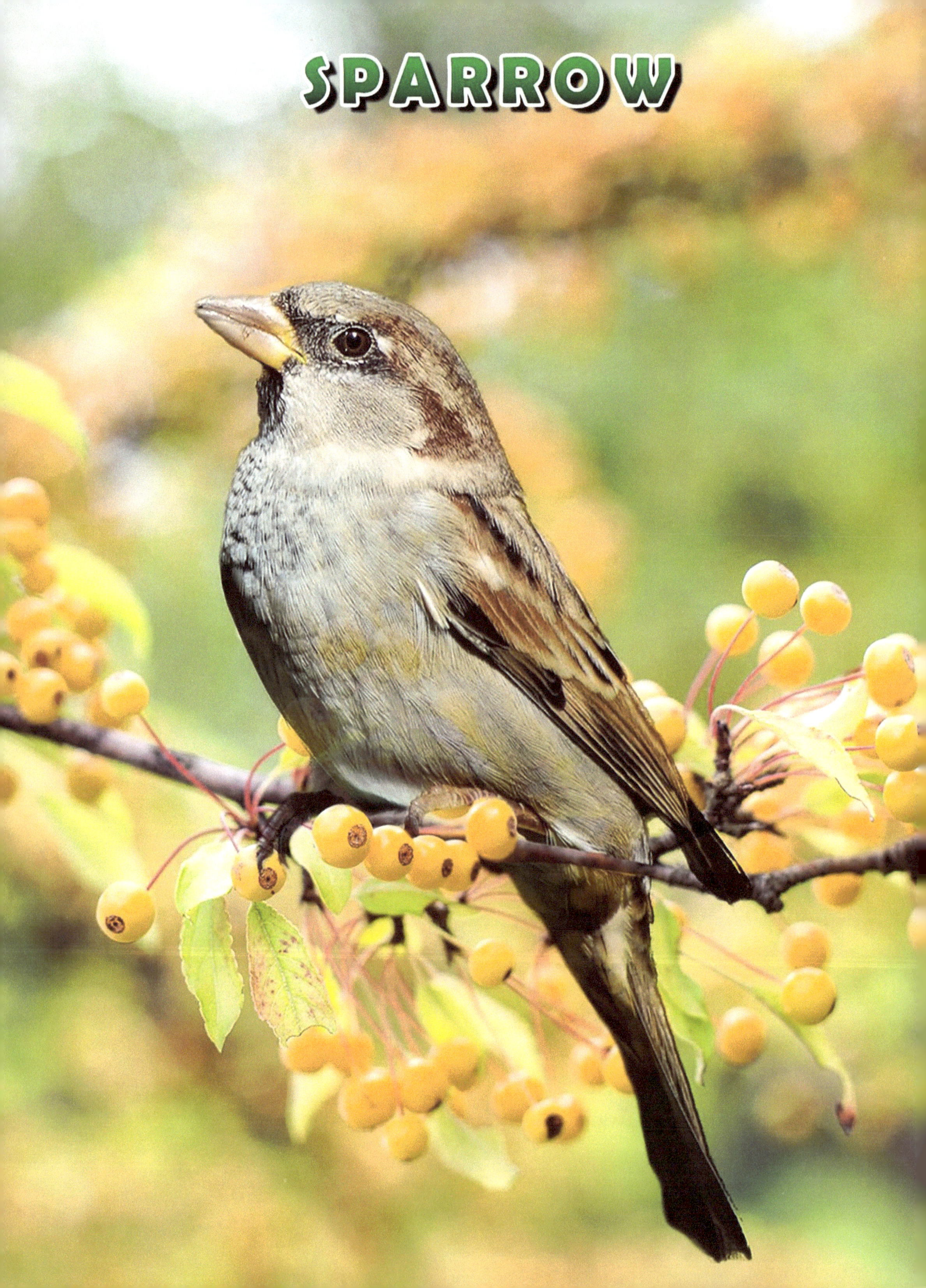

STORK

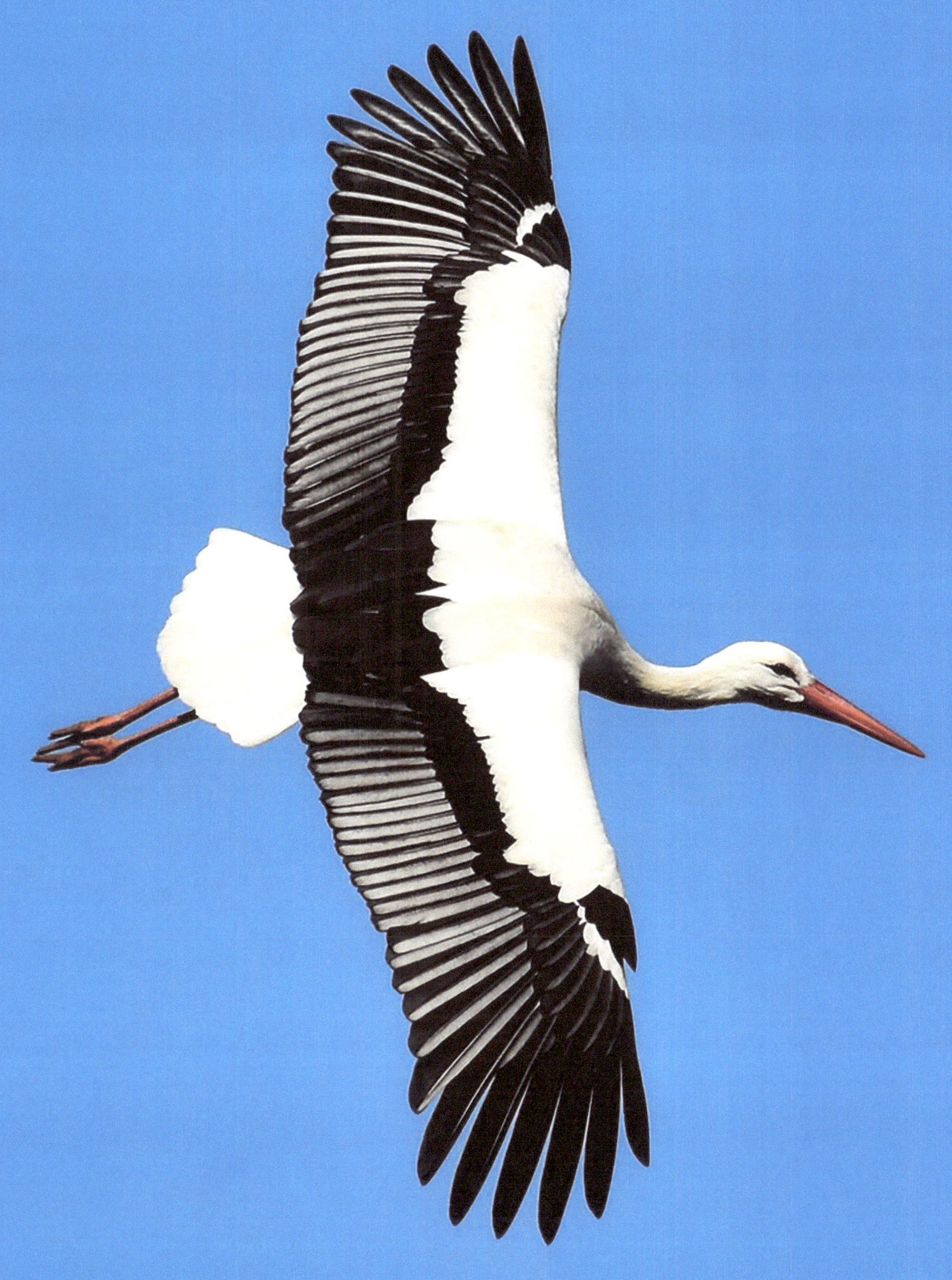

SWALLOWS

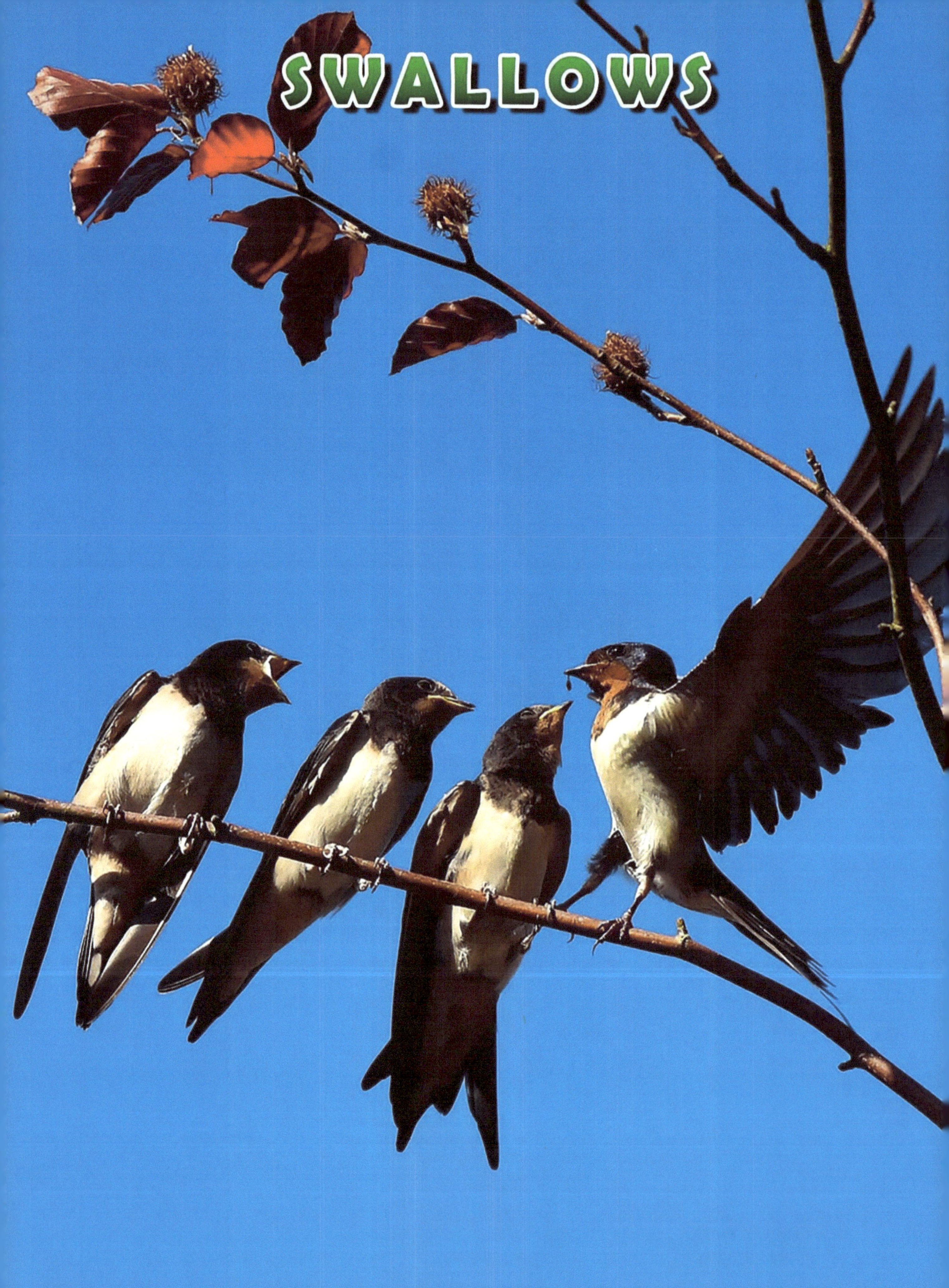

TANAGER

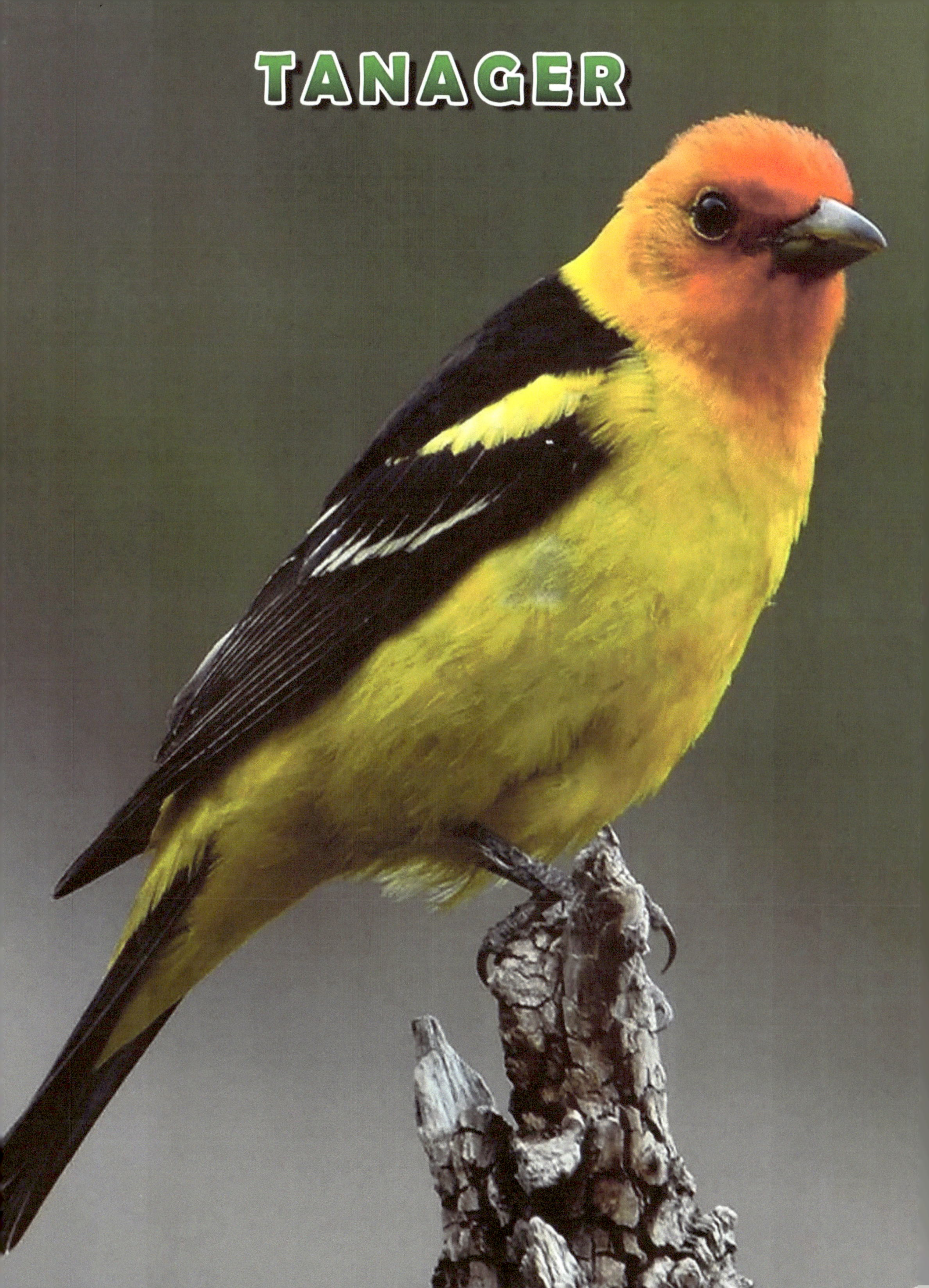

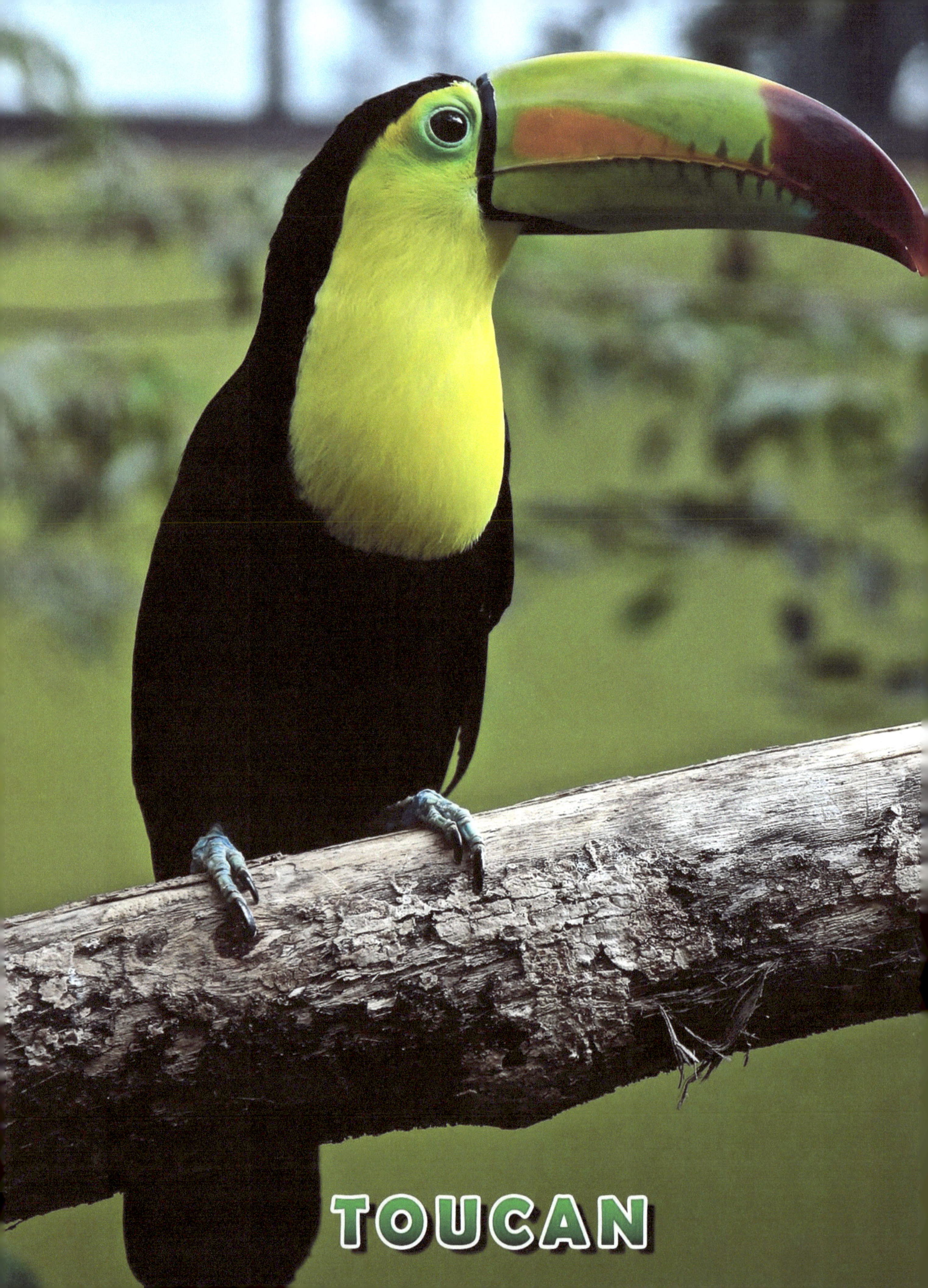

TOUCAN

TURACO

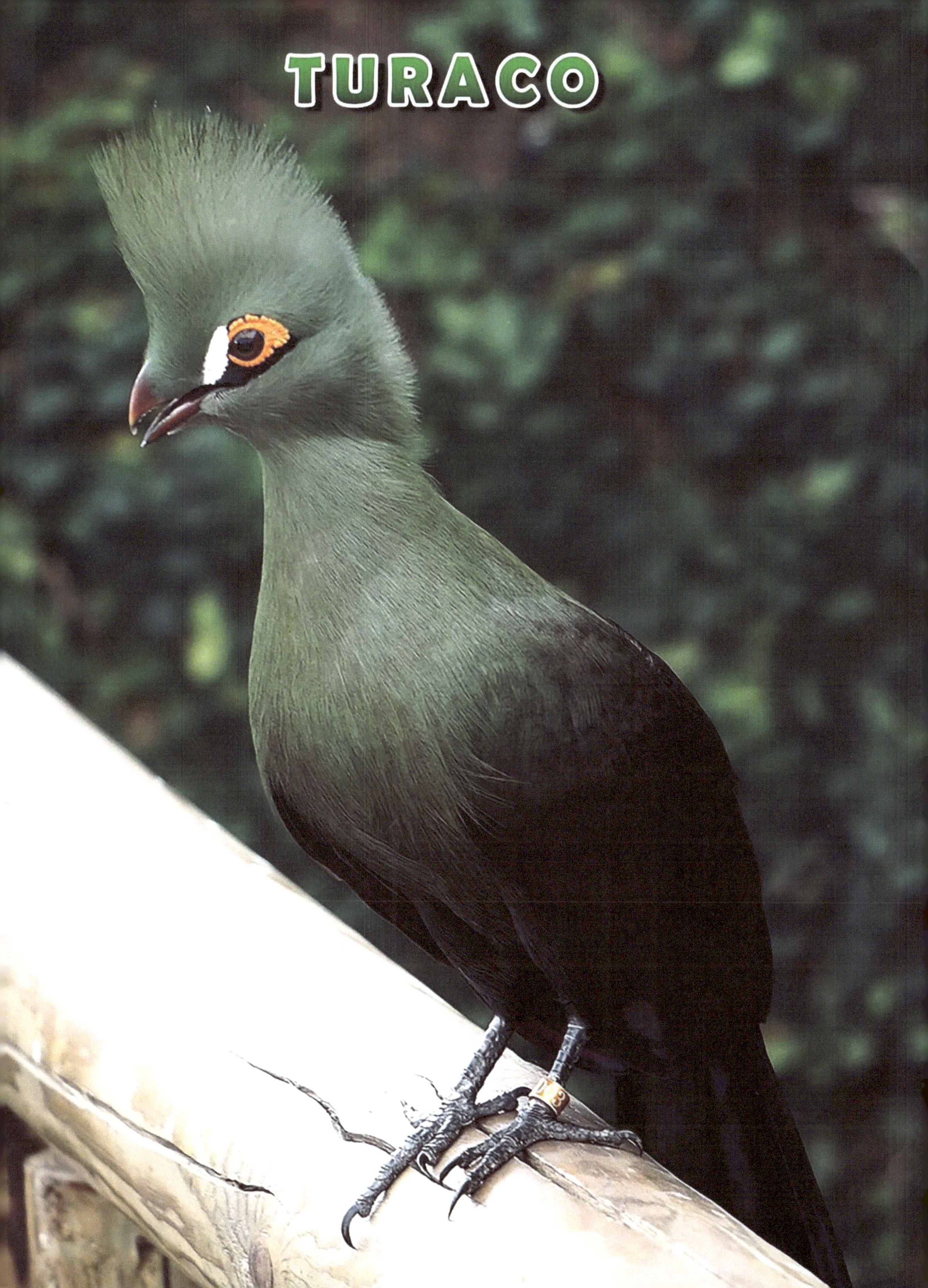

WAXWING

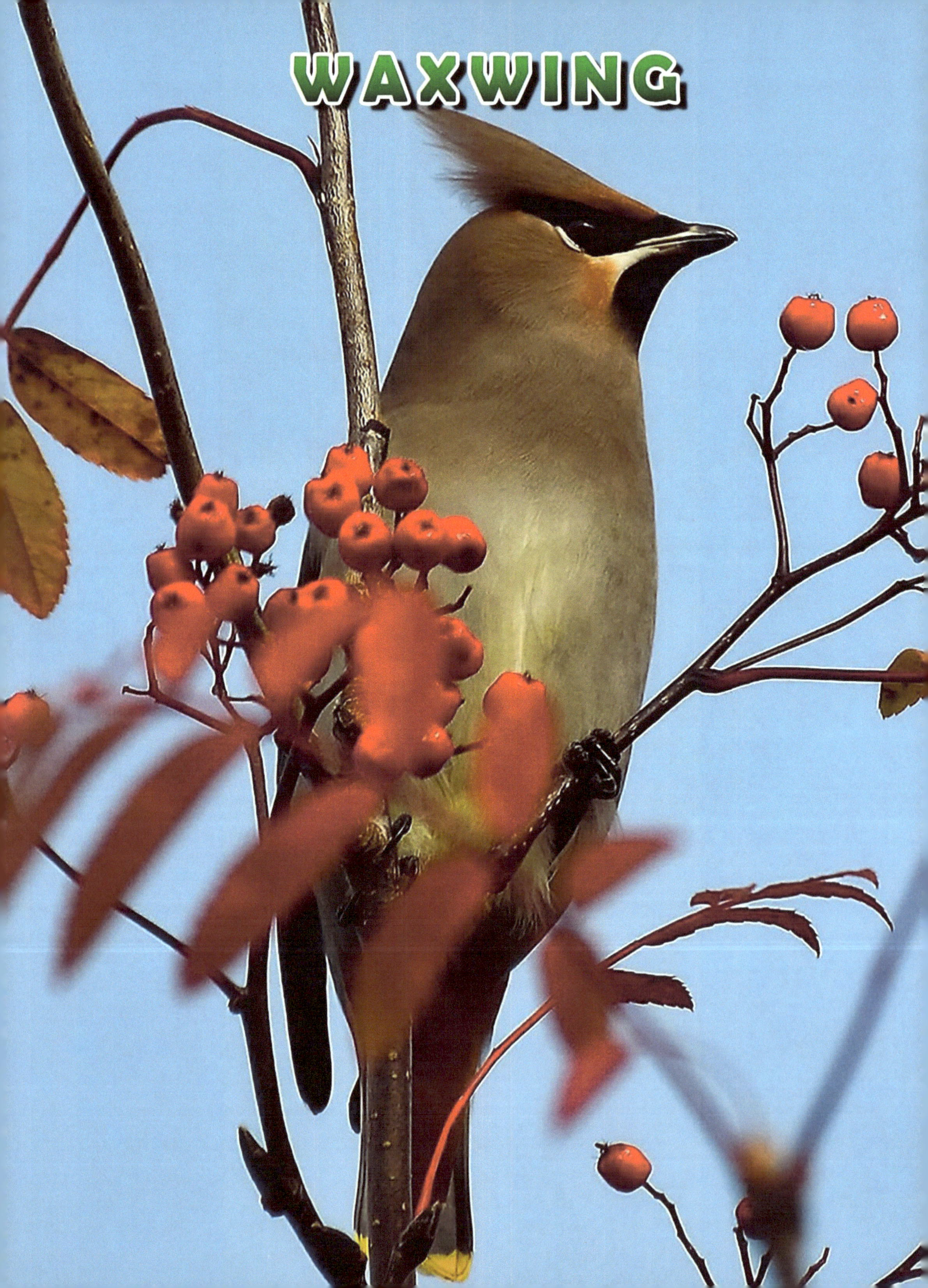

WREN

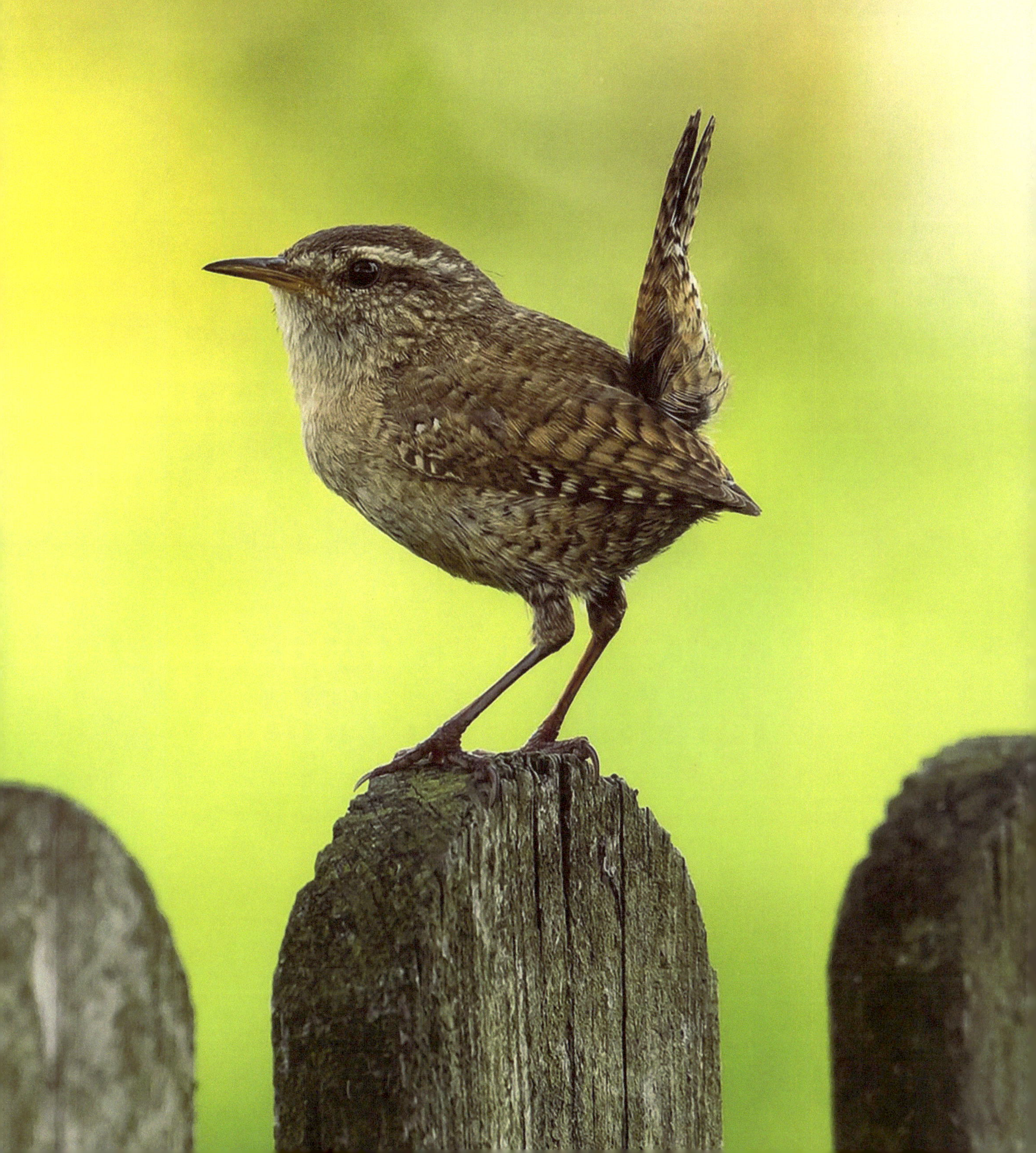

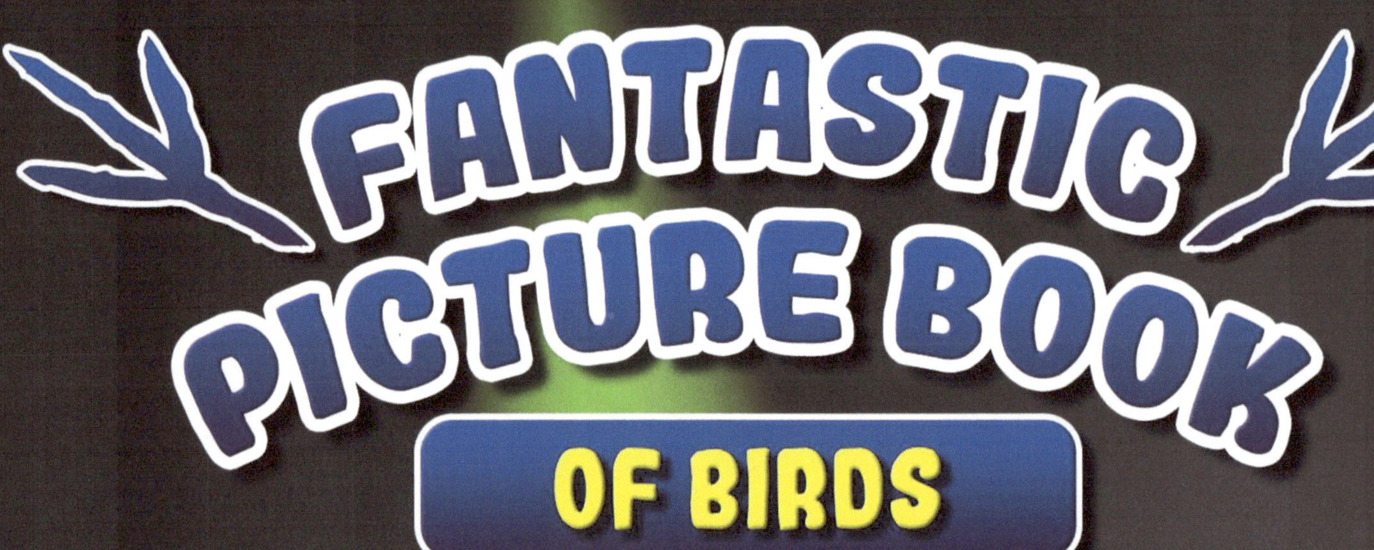

THANK YOU FOR BUYING.

If you have enjoyed this book, please tell your friends.

For more books, please visit: etidbitz.com/books

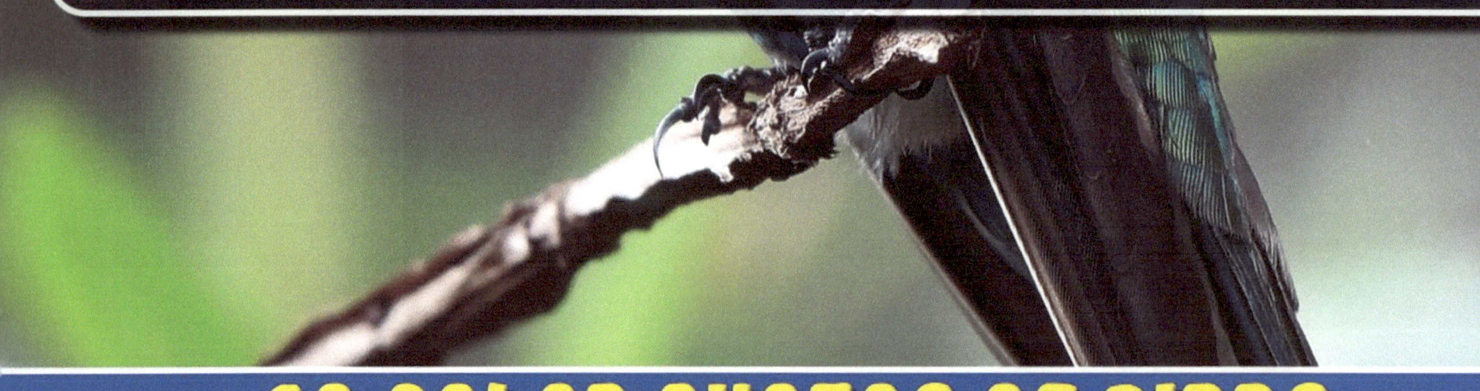